TABLE OF CONTENTS

TABLE OF CONTENTS (CON'T)

PART 3 :: MIND: YOUR THOUGHTS CREATE YOUR REALITY

INTRODUCTION

MY STORY

I wasn't always that interested in the foods that I ate, how I moved my body, or even the thoughts that floated around in my mind. They were just there. Looking back, it was almost as though I was just going through the motions of living life. Growing up, home-cooked meals were a staple in our household—my grandmother lived with us and I remember always having food made from "scratch"—but we did have our fair share of processed foods as well.

High school and college were a free-for-all. I don't think I ever used the stove, not once. It was years of takeout, pub food, pizza and wings, not to mention copious amounts of the alcohol paired with the drug du jour and about a pack of cigarettes a day. I didn't work out at all; I was way to busy having a good time. I went out all night and slept all day, in between classes of course. I do remember being extremely unhappy with how I looked and felt, but didn't really know how to change it.

For as long as I can remember, I always had an issue with my body. I wasn't ever really overweight, but in my mind my thighs were too big, I was way too flabby everywhere, and I always needed to lose ten or fifteen pounds.

As soon as my clothes would start to get tight, I would jump on the low-fat bandwagon, but mostly I would just skip meals altogether. I would hit the gym and run like Forrest Gump on the treadmill until my jeans got loose again. This cycle lasted for years, and then I got pregnant...with twins...and gained seventy pounds!

I dieted like crazy for a year after giving birth to my first two daughters, and I lost most of the weight, but I was skinny-fat. I cooked and ate home-cooked meals, but I still bought processed foods. My eating was all over the place. It was after my second pregnancy that I knew I had to change something.

> I thought I was making healthy food choices. I really didn't think there was anything wrong with the way I ate.

I thought I was making healthy food choices. I really didn't think there was anything wrong with the way I ate. In fact, because I was preparing most of my foods at home, I was convinced that my diet was pretty darn good. I was young and I was healthy. I did everything right—or so I thought, until I felt that lump that wouldn't go away in November 2007.

It was also around this time that I committed to joining a gym and, through a friend, was introduced to CrossFit. After fifteen years I finally quit smoking. I was active, excited, and feeling great. I started learning about nutrition and how what I ate affected my body. I was loving the change, but that lump kept growing.

I kept being told not to worry; that women, especially young women, have lumpy breasts; and after many doctors' visits, numerous ultrasounds, and even a biopsy that came back negative, I finally listened to that nagging feeling in my gut and asked that it be removed. In August of 2008, I had a lumpectomy. It was finally gone!

Two week later, in September, at thirty-two years old, I was diagnosed with Invasive Ductal Carcinoma In Situ and was immediately told I would need a mastectomy, chemotherapy and radiation followed by five to ten years of hormone therapy.

I had a million questions and not enough answers. Needless to say, I was overwhelmed.

I went into full-on, lockdown research mode. I scoured the internet, bought every book on cancer that I could find. I saw every naturopath, oncologist, radiologist, plastic surgeon, and reconstructive surgeon in the city. I went to fake boob shops, I went to lingerie stores and tried on "special" bras—found some really nice ones!

Aside from my treatments, one of my biggest concerns was whether or not I would be able to work out after my surgeries. I couldn't find anyone in my situation who was young and fit and who trained like I did and who had cancer! I was told I wouldn't be able to lift five pounds over my head again.

I was also told that what I ate had no effect on my diagnosis. This, more than anything, just didn't sit right with me. Again, that feeling in my gut told me otherwise.

I decided to have the mastectomy, and I did the chemotherapy, which almost killed me. It was the worst six months of my life.

When it was time for radiation, though, I had had enough. I made a decision and refused radiation and Tamoxifan.

> What I ate, how much and how often I moved, and how my thoughts, both negative and positive, affected all of my actions now became a priority.

Somewhere halfway through my treatments, my thoughts shifted from killing cancer to healing my body. Before my chemo began, I had started eating a Paleo diet. It wasn't perfect, but I was learning. I was still hanging on to my old familiar habits, but there came a point where I realized that in order to move forward and save my life, I had to change everything.

What I ate, how much and how often I moved, and how my thoughts, both negative and positive, affected all of my actions now became a priority. I got rid of all the alcohol, all the drugs, all the toxins in my life—including unhealthy relationships—and focused on healing my body.

Eating a strict Paleo diet was now a priority. During that first year and to this day, I intermittently go ketogenic for a period of time ("Ketogenic" means I remove all sugars from my diet and focus on protein and fats for energy) to reset.

What I did notice through my treatments was that despite all the poison they were putting in my body, I was thriving. I was strong! My blood counts were always stable and my doctors were always surprised at how well my body tolerated the treatments. I wasn't the status quo!

I knew that my approach was working. I knew that the foods I was eating were nourishing my body; they were healing my cancer. I knew that my training was helping me to build a strong foundation. My body was thriving.

Five years later, having experienced the benefits of my lifestyle changes firsthand, I want to share all of this with you. Not only am I living cancer free, I now no longer worry about how I look, think how big my thighs are, or obsess over ten pounds. I instead focus on how I feel when I'm filling up on the good stuff. I don't crave junk foods any longer; I crave foods that nourish my body. I crave movement that makes me feel alive, and I focus on creating loving relationships that support and empower me. The thing is, you don't need to be told that you might die to start living. You just have to want to take that first step.

A better, stronger, healthier life all begins with a choice, a choice to start living the best version of you. Let me show you how!

PART 1 :: NUTRITION - YOU ARE WHAT YOU EAT!

1.1 GETTING HEALTHY!

Have you ever thought about why we have time for everything in our lives except to feed ourselves properly? We can spend hours upon hours in front of the TV, or on Facebook or Twitter, but then find it exceedingly difficult to prepare good meals. Everything around us today is built upon convenience

A healthy body performs and works at its optimum, has the ability to fight off illness, and can keep you strong and give you energy all day long. Being healthy gets you going. You feel amazing in your skin, you wake up in the morning energized and ready to start your day. Your mind is clear and focused and your thoughts are in line with who you are.

If you're healthy, amazing. Keep learning and doing what you feel is optimal for you. If you're not healthy, you must do whatever you can to give every cell in your body the support it needs to build a strong immune system. The foods that you eat should make you healthy!

1.2 THE PALEO PLAN

So what is the Paleo diet? The term often brings up images of cavewomen roaming the fields for fresh leafy greens, picking berries with their babies strapped to their backs, and cavemen, spears in hand, hunting for their next kill. And that may have been true millions of years ago! Modern-day Paleo is, of course, far removed from our spear-throwing ancestors, but some principles have remained the same.

Paleo eating (let's take the word "diet' out of the equation) means eating REAL FOODS that are whole and unprocessed, foods that actually have a shelf life shorter than our attention spans! It is about obtaining the best-quality foods available to us and that will provide the most nutrients to nourish our bodies at a cellular level. It's about helping our bodies thrive, and healing them from the damage of our modern-day food system. It involves eating healthy, fresh, and live foods. This means seasonal fruits and vegetables, lean meats from quality sources, and good fats. The human body has not only evolved but thrived over the last two million years eating this way.

For most of human history, we have survived eating foods we have found in nature. The evolution of our current diet came along with the Neolithic or Agricultural Revolution a mere ten thousand years ago—not enough time has passed for our bodies to adapt to eating modern foods.

Paleo eating (let's take the word "diet" out of the equation) means eating REAL FOODS that are whole and unprocessed... It is about obtaining the best-quality foods available to us

The Industrial Revolution, only two hundred years old, has added another dimension. We have changed our dietary habits more in the last two hundred years than all of humanity has in the previous hundred thousand. Our grocery stores and food supply are now filled with more simple sugars, refined foods, processed foods, and foods filled with chemicals than ever before. Our bodies are not adapted to eating this way, and we are starting to see the effects of our poor food choices. Food intolerances are more frequent and quickly becoming the norm. Modern-day diseases such as autoimmune disorders, cancer, diabetes, obesity, and cardiovascular disease are rampant.

The Paleo approach brings us back to eating the most nutrient-dense foods possible. It's an approach to building a strong, healthy body by reducing inflammation and getting rid of toxins that are found in most of the foods we eat today. Yes, it's a way of eating that mimics our hunter-gatherer ancestors with a balance of lean meats, seafood, vegetables, fruit, and some nuts and seeds, but don't get caught up in the words *Paleo* or *Primal* and think that unless you're chewing raw meat off a bone you're doing it wrong.

It's not a dogmatic approach, and it's not a diet. Instead, it's a framework that will help you get healthy and give your body what it needs to function at its best, exactly as it was meant to.

As the Paleo lifestyle becomes more mainstream (and it has—even Dr. Oz is talking about it now), **there are a lot of questions and differing opinions on what actually constitutes Paleo. Is it low carb or high carb? Does all dairy have to be removed? How about grains...do they all have to go?**

There are some diehards who wouldn't even consider veering off the Paleolithic path, and others who occasionally enjoy some sushi *with* the rice on a Friday night.

How you approach Paleo eating depends on your perspective, your needs, and your goals. There is no one-size-fits-all solution; our bodies all adapt and react to foods differently.

Paleo is best viewed as a template, a starting place. If you have autoimmune issues, it may be a good idea to remove nightshades from your diet; if you're an athlete it's important that you eating enough carbs, so you may want to include some starchy white rice; if you're trying to lose weight, you may want to minimize fruit, and if you have cancer, dairy is out!

The goal of creating a lifestyle based on the Paleolithic framework is to ultimately eat foods that maximize nutrient density and promote health and remove those that wreak havoc on our metabolic, digestive, and immune systems.

People who have adopted a Paleo approach to eating have seen significant results in health, body composition, and energy levels, and often in record time.

It makes people feel better. It allows us to heal our bodies from the onslaught of toxins and chemicals we have grown accustomed to. Athletes follow it for optimal performance, those with health issues see amazing changes, often reversing symptoms completely; people effortlessly lose weight, gain muscle, and have more energy. Inflammation, the root cause of so many diseases, is reduced. Digestive problems and allergies often disappear. We look and feel younger, and, most importantly, we are healthier.

There are very few things that impact your life as powerfully as changing the foods you eat.

And the food tastes fantastic. Our taste buds have been so accustomed to salty, sugary, and chemically enhanced foods that we've forgotten how good real food tastes. Once you reunite your taste buds with the natural tastes of fresh veggies, herbs, and spices, you will be so surprised at how much you enjoy them.

There are very few things that impact your life as powerfully as changing the foods you eat. Within hours, whatever you put into your mouth is replacing cells in your body. Every piece of food that you consume has a direct impact on your body, your mind, and your spirit. Doesn't it make sense, then, to fill your body with the best foods available—foods that make you healthy and thriving?

THE PRINCIPLES ARE SIMPLE:

- **Eat foods that create health.**

  Real, whole foods. This includes foods that are organic, un-processed, and unrefined. They are foods that are prepared as close to their natural state as possible. They do not have added ingredients. Nothing compares to Mother Nature's garden. I always say if your great-grandmother wouldn't have grown it, eaten, it or recognized it, don't eat it! Fill your body with the vitamins, minerals, cancer-fighting phyto-chemicals, and antioxidants that enrich your health.

  > If your great-grandmother wouldn't have grown it, eaten, it or recognized it, don't eat it!

- **Avoid foods that cheat you of your health.**

  Toxic foods. I encourage you to reduce or eliminate all foods that create inflammation in your body. Inflammation drastically reduces the quality of your life. It sucks the energy right out of you, creates chronic disease, and weakens your immune system. It just plain sucks! Cancer, heart disease, Alzheimer's, and autoimmune issues have all been linked to inflammatory responses in the body. It's also a major cause of weight gain and weight-loss resistance. Oddly enough, many of the foods recommended by the standard North American diet are composed of foods that irritate our bodies. Grains, legumes, dairy, sugar, trans fats, processed foods, and anything that comes in a box, container, jar or bottle are part of that list. Unless you shop the perimeter of the grocery store, you're most likely buying processed foods. Removing foods that contain sugars, additives, preservatives, table salt, and excess fats is a must. If you can't understand the wording on the label, don't eat it! In fact, it's best if it doesn't have a label!!

- **Keep it simple.**
Counting calories and weighing your food is not fun. I've done it and I don't like it. Eating should be about enjoyment! Having a healthy relationship with your food creates a strong foundation and a basis for a lifestyle that you can sustain and celebrate. And believe me when I say that the more you fill up on the good stuff, the less junk you'll want. You will start to listen to your body again, and understand what it needs and what it doesn't. You'll start to regain that energy you had long ago, you'll look better, you'll feel better, and, most importantly you'll find that connection with yourself.

- **Enjoy!**
As a mom to three kiddos, I know that creating meals from scratch can feel daunting and really time consuming. Make mealtime fun. It doesn't have to be a process and it doesn't have to be complicated. Nutritious and healthy meals can be simple and fast.

1.3 PROTEIN IS STRENGTH

Protein makes up part of the structure of every cell, tissue, and organ in your body. The protein you eat is broken down into amino acids, which are responsible for pretty much every biochemical reaction that your body has, from breathing to digesting your food to running a marathon. Hormones, neurotransmitters, enzymes, and even your DNA are made up of amino acids. They are the building blocks of life and also the stepping stones to recovery. They influence every system in the body.

Lean and clean proteins balance the effects of insulin-promoting weight loss, preventing insulin resistance and majorly benefitting your metabolism. They also help satisfy your appetite. If weight loss isn't your goal, eating enough protein provides a balance of energy levels throughout the day.

Can't focus? Eating protein helps to stimulate clearer thinking; it's the building block of your brain's network. Need to get strong? It's the best way to build muscle and repair tissue. It's also what gives us great skin, hair, and nails!

Paleo foods emphasize complete proteins. There are twenty amino acids needed to make a protein. Your body can formulate two thirds on its own, and you must get the other eight essential amino acids from the foods you eat. A complete protein is one that contains all of the essential amino acids, and is always found in animal-based foods, including meat, poultry, seafood, eggs, and dairy.

EXCELLENT SOURCES OF PROTEIN

EGGS	OSTRICH	MACKAREL
BEEF	PORK	MAHI MAHI
BISON	QUAIL	MUSSELS
BOAR	RABBIT	OYSTERS
BUFFALO	TURKEY	SALMON
CHICKEN	VEAL	SARDINES
DUCK	VENISON	SCALLOPS
GAME MEATS	CARP	SHRIMP
GOAT	CLAMS	SNAIL
GOOSE	GROUPER	SNAPPER
LAMB	HALIBUT	SWORDFISH
MUTTON	HERRING	TROUT
ORGAN MEATS	LOBSTER	TUNA

Eating quality proteins is a critical part of an optimal diet.

On the other hand, an incomplete protein source is one that only provides some of the essential amino acids. Foods like whole grains, beans, nuts, seeds, peas, and corn are considered incomplete proteins. Most vegetarians have to combine these foods or supplement to get the complete spectrum of amino acids needed. Also, many of these foods happen to be gut-irritating. They contain high amounts of lectins and phytates, which challenge your immune system and interfere with the absorption of many important vitamins and minerals. Eating clean animal proteins is an important part of a healthy diet. This means sourcing your foods and getting the best-quality grassfed meats, wild fish, and free-range chickens that are available to you.

GROUND RULES AND GUIDELINES FOR PROTEIN

Focus on eating the **best-quality meats** you can get your hands on. Grass-fed meats, wild game, hormone- and antibiotic-free chickens and turkey, and wild fish are ideal. They are free of hormones, antibiotics, pesticides, and chemical residues.

If conventional meats are your only option, buy lean cuts of meat. Hormones and toxins are typically stored in fat tissue. If you're eating an animal that has been exposed to eating poor-quality foods like corn or soy, you can bet that you are eating that same corn or soy.

Stay away from farmed fish. They, too, are full of toxins. They have concentrations of antibiotics and pesticides, are fattier and therefore store toxins more readily, are imbalanced in Omega 3 and Omega 6 fats, which creates inflammation in the body, have a lower protein content than their wild caught counterparts, and are less healthy nutritionally.

HOW MUCH PROTEIN?

Everyone is talking about getting enough protein, but what does that look like? Protein requirements are based on body weight and activity level.

The basic recommendation is 0.8 grams per kilogram of body weight daily for the average healthy adult. For example, a 140-pound woman would need to consume around 51 grams a day.

> The amount of protein each of us needs is a bit different.

If you're an athlete, you're going to need more protein, because your body is constantly building and repairing muscle. Most experts recommend an intake in the range of 1.2–2.0 g/kg (or around .54g-.9g/lb). Using the same example of a 140-pound woman, she would then need around 75-126g of protein per day. Some experts recommend as much as 1 gram per pound of body for higher-intensity work.

BE A LABEL NINJA. KNOW YOUR LABELS.

Marketing has done an amazing job at confusing consumers as to what they're purchasing when in comes to buying meat and poultry. Here's a list of what you should look out for.

KNOW YOUR LABELS

• PASTURED

This means the animal was allowed to forage freely as it was meant to, feeding on grasses and seeds and insects. There is no restriction from the outdoors. The animal may have been fed grains by the farmer, especially in the winter, if the farm is in a cold climate.

• GRASS-FED

Grass-fed means that the animal was fed on the food it evolved to eat, which is grass, and has eaten little or no grain. Sometimes an animal is "finished" on grains, meaning it ate grain during the last two to three months of its life. If you're looking for no grains, select 100% grass-fed.

• ORGANIC

This means that the meat or eggs are required to come from animals that have been solely fed organic feed. They are also not allowed to receive antibiotics or hormones of any kind. "Organic" is the only label of the list that is regulated with inspections and enforcement.

• OMEGA 3 ENRICHED

These are claims that the animal has been fed a diet rich in Omega 3 fatty acids.

• FREE RANGE

Animals must have access to the outdoors. There is no specification as to quality or duration of that outside exposure. Some farmers allow their animals to roam freely; others may provide an access door or an open window that leads to an area of dirt space. It is better option than cage-free.

• NATURALLY RAISED

A regulated term meaning the animals have been raised without the use antibiotics, added growth hormones, or animal by-products. It does not regulate the welfare of the animal or what it eats.

• CAGE-FREE

This simply means that the chickens are not kept in cages; they are allowed to roam freely in their henhouse. They have little or no access to the outdoors.

KNOW YOUR LABELS (CON'T)

• VEGETARIAN RAISED

This is a newer term, and means the farmer didn't feed the animals any meat, fish, or animal by-products. Usually used with chickens and eggs and is a bit deceiving, as chickens are carnivores and will eat bugs and insects on their own when allowed to forage freely. A chicken raised on vegetarian feed has been raised solely on industrialized feed, usually GMO grains.

• NATURAL

Means that during processing, nothing synthetic is added to the meat. The guidelines do not prohibit the use of antibiotics, growth hormones, or animal byproducts.

1.4 TO CARB OR NOT TO CARB

Our bodies do not actually need carbohydrates—we can live without them, but our energy levels will definitely suffer. Carbohydrates give your body the fuel that it needs to support a healthy life. Carbs have also been hotly debated because of the many diet crazes that have created confusion surrounding how much and which carbs you should be eating. Low carb, high carb, no carb—sound familiar?

The important thing is the type of carbohydrate you choose to eat.

There are two types: complex carbohydrates, which are found in vegetables and fruits, whole grains, and legumes (grains and legumes, FYI, are not considered Paleo—more on that later), and simple carbohydrates, which are found in sugary junk foods and refined grain products like breads and pastas.

Most of what you eat should come from complex carbs. Eating this way will allow a slow and steady supply of energy to your body and brain and help you to stay focused and full of energy. Complex carbs are typically higher in fiber, which means their sugars are released more slowly into the bloodstream, keeping you feeling fuller longer and minimizing any insulin spikes.

It's not about avoiding carbohydrates, it's about choosing the right carbohydrates.

Simple carbs provide empty calories. They are stripped of any nutritional value and always leave you wanting more. Ever notice how you can eat an endless supply of potato chips or a plate of pasta and not feel full, then get tired right after and be hungry again a short time after that? These foods really do a number on your insulin levels, they promote inflammation within your body, and create an environment that supports all kinds of issues like leaky gut, autoimmune disorders, weight issues, diabetes, and obesity, just to name a few.

Paleo eating focuses on getting your carbohydrates from whole food sources, live foods, vegetables and fruits, and non-toxic foods, creating a lifestyle that supports your body. It's not about avoiding carbohydrates, it's about choosing the right carbohydrates. Your food should make you healthy!

CARBS THAT HELP ME THRIVE

Your first focus should be on eating non-starchy veggies. Walk the perimeter of the grocery store or visit your local famers' market and stock up on these amazing nutrient-dense foods. There are so many options. They are full of antioxidants, which help lower oxidative stress and reduce inflammation. They are packed with vitamins and minerals, and are an amazing source of fiber. Don't be shy, load your plate with plants!

NON-STARCHY VEGGIES

ARTICHOKE	COLLARD GREENS	ONIONS
ASPARAGUS	CUCUMBERS	PARSLEY
ARUGULA	EGGPLANT	RADICCHIO
BAMBOO SHOOTS	ENDIVE	RADISHES
BEET GREENS	FENNEL	SHALLOTS
BELL PEPPERS	GARLIC	SPINACH
BOK CHOY	GREEN BEANS	SWISS CHARD
BROCCOLI,	KALE	TURNIP GREENS
BROCCOLINI	KOHLRABI	WATERCRESS
BRUSSELS SPROUTS	LEEKS	ZUCCHINI
CABBAGE	LETTUCE	
CAULIFLOWER	MUSHROOMS	
CELERY	MUSTARD GREENS	

Next, you want to focus on veggies that are higher in starch, and fruits. Both non-starchy and starchy vegetables are an important part of what you eat. The major difference between the two is starch content; higher starch means these foods are also higher in calories and carbs. They are, however, both packed with tons of fiber, vitamins and minerals, and are still overall relatively low in calories. They are usually found in root vegetables.

STARCHY VEGGIES

BEETS	PLANTAINS
CARROTS	PUMPKINS
CHESTNUTS	SPLIT PEAS
JICAMA	SWEET POTATOES/YAMS
OKRA	SQUASH (ACORN, BUTTERNUT, WINTER)
PARSNIPS	TOMATOES
POTATOES	TURNIP

A NOTE ON NIGHTSHADES

Nightshades can be a problem food for some. Eggplants, peppers, tomatoes, and potatoes are part of the nightshade family, and are known to cause issues with autoimmunity. Like grains and legumes, they contain lectins (a protein found in many foods) that can trigger an autoimmune response in the body. It is most often connected to joint pain, arthritis, Type 1 diabetes, and celiac disease. Pay attention to how you feel after eating these. Eliminating them from your diet for a period of time to see if you have any sensitivities may be worth the experiment.

FRUITS

Fruits, like vegetables, are an amazing source of essential antioxidants, vitamins and minerals, phytonutrients, and fiber. They will make you healthy! They are, how-

ALL-STAR FRUIT OPTIONS

BLACKBERRIES
BLUEBERRIES
ELDERBERRIES
GOOSEBERRIES
STRAWBERRIES
RASPBERRIES

ever, also loaded with natural sugars–their sweetness is why we love them. **Eat fruit, but don't make it the star of the show.** Veggies always trump any fruit you eat during a meal. And please ditch the fruit juice and fruit smoothies, you might as well be eating a Snickers bar! Start with one to two servings of fresh whole fruits per day.

FRUITS (CON'T)

NEXT BEST OPTIONS

APPLES
APRICOTS
CHERRIES
GRAPEFRUIT
KIWI
LEMONS
LIMES
MELONS
ORANGES/NECTARINES/TANGERINES
PEACHES
PEARS
PLUMS
POMEGRANATES

EAT IN MODERATION

BANANAS
GRAPES
MANGO
PAPAYA
PINEAPPLE
WATERMELON

DIRTY DOZEN, CLEAN FIFTEEN

As often as you can, try and buy organic fruits and vegetables. Conventional produce is usually very heavily sprayed with pesticides. The EWG (Environmental Working Group) has a list of fruits and vegetables that it classifies as the "dirtiest," being the most contaminated to the "cleanest," or the least contaminated. Go local and buy your produce in season as often as possible.

If budget is an issue, try and at least purchase organic for the top dirty foods on the list.

1.5 FAT IS YOUR FRIEND

There is no way around this one: if you want to be healthy, you have to eat fat. It reduces inflammation, helps your body absorb vitamins, fuels your body throughout the day, and keeps your hair and skin glowing. You even need to eat fat to burn fat. Fat has gotten such a bad rap over the last twenty or thirty years, though, that everyone is afraid to eat it.

What is important to know is that fat is essential, and that not every fat is created equal. You have to focus on eating the good fats, eliminate the wrong ones, and create a good balance between mono- and polyunsaturated fats (Omegas 3s and 6s).

THE FATS YOU NEED TO FOCUS ON

Saturated Fats

COCONUT OIL
PALM OIL
LARD

THE FATS YOU NEED TO FOCUS ON (CON'T)

TALLOW
BUTTER
GHEE
DUCK
GOOSE
CHICKEN
WILD COLD WATER FISH

UNSATURATED FATS

AVOCADO*
OLIVE OIL, OLIVES*
RAW NUTS AND NUT BUTTERS (NO PEANUTS)
RAW SEEDS
FLAX OIL**

*unsaturated fats are typically not your best options for cooking, as they are easily oxidized and are unstable at high temperatures. Drizzle freely on your salads and opt for more stable forms of fat when cooking.

**flaxseed oil is often promoted as a great way to get Omega 3s, but your body does not convert flax very efficiently, and supplementing with too much of it may throw off your Omega 3/Omega 6 balance.

Wait...that list says "Saturated"! I thought saturated fats were bad for me!

This has become so wildly accepted that people have, out of fear, stopped eating what is in fact good for them. In their pursuit of health and weight loss, we've started buying low-fat versions of everything,

What is important to know is that fat is essential, and that not every fat is created equal.

ditched egg yolks and made pretty much every type of meat the
bad guy.

Saturated fat is not bad for you. If it comes from high-quality
sources, it can actually make you healthier. And it doesn't cause
heart disease! It unfortunately got a bad rap from a study done by
Ancel Keys in the 1950s that blamed dietary fats for clogging arter-
ies and promoting heart disease. That study alone changed the way
the whole world viewed saturated fats. It has since, however, been
proven flawed.

THE FATS YOU NEED TO GET RID OF

ANY MAN-MADE OR PROCESSED FATS, ESPECIALLY TRANS FATS
MARGARINE
HYDROGENATED OILS
CANOLA OIL
VEGETABLE OIL
SOYBEAN OIL
CORN OIL
GRAPESEED OIL
SUNFLOWER OIL
SAFFLOWER OIL

The *Journal of Clinical Nutrition* in 2010 published a massive
study that concluded there is not enough evidence to suggest saturated fats and cholesterol cause heart disease. The body loves

fat, but from sources like grass-fed meats, butter, whole eggs (yes, with the yolk), and coconut fat, not Chinese food and pizza. Just make sure your sources are healthy ones.

MUFAS AND PUFAS: A LOVE-FAT RELATIONSHIP

There are two kinds of unsaturated fats: monounsaturated and polyunsaturated. They are primarily found in vegetable oils and in nuts and seeds.

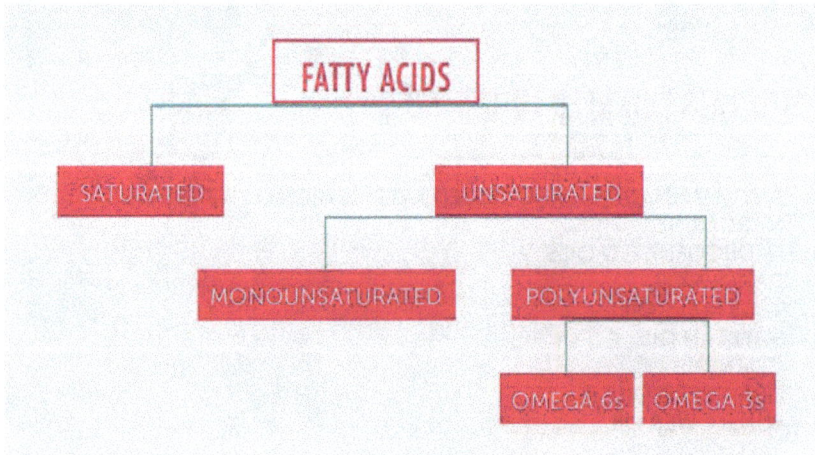

Monounsaturated fats are liquid at room temperature but solidify at cold temperatures. The richest sources include olive, rapeseed, hazelnut, and almond oils, avocados, olives, nuts, and seeds. They are thought to have the greatest health benefits. They reduce total cholesterol, specifically LDL cholesterol without affecting HDL cholesterol.

Polyunsaturated fats are always liquid, in both room and cold temperatures. Sources include most vegetable oils and oily fish. They reduce LDL blood levels; however, they can also reduce HDL cholesterol.

It is a good idea to replace some of your polyunsaturated fats with monounsaturated ones.

THE OMEGAS

I'm sure you've all heard about Omega 3s and Omega 6s by now. In case you haven't, these two essential fatty acids are sub-groups of polyunsaturated fats. They cannot be made by the body and have to come from food sources.

Omega 3s can further be divided into 3 groups: ALA, EPA, and DHA. Studies show that the people with the highest intake of Omega 3 fatty acids have a lower risk of heart attacks. Omega 6s are important for the healthy functioning of cell membranes; they make your skin super healthy.

The absolute best sources of Omega 3s can be found in wild-caught oily fish like fresh tuna or salmon, sardines, and mackerel, and their fish oils.

The richest plant sources are flaxseed and oil, pumpkin seeds, walnuts, rapeseed oil, and soybeans. (Stay away from soy; the majority is GMO.)

Animal sources are available to your body right away; plant sources need to be converted.

We need both Omegas to thrive in the right ratios.

Over the last hundred years or so there has been a dramatic increase in our modern diets in the ratio of Omega 6 and Omega 3 fats. There has to be the right balance to achieve optimal health.

Today, our diets are consistently richer in Omega 6 fats as compared to our ancestors. They ate a lot more fish and seafood and a lot fewer seed oils. The industrial revolution introduced vegetable oils and cereal grains in abundance. Way more Omega 6s, a lot fewer Omega 3s.

More of one is not better without less of the other. Make sure to add more Omega 3s to your diet. Choose your fats wisely!

OIL	OMEGA-3	OMEGA-6
SAFFLOWER	0%	75%
SUNFLOWER	0%	65%
CORN	0%	54%
COTTONSEED	0%	50%
SESAME	0%	42%
PEANUT	0%	32%
SOYBEAN	7%	51%
CANOLA	9%	20%
WALNUT	10%	52%
FLAXSEED	57%	14%
FISH	100%	0%

1.6 LESS HEALTHY FOODS

GRAINS: YES, YOU CAN SURVIVE WITHOUT THEM!

What do you mean, no cereal or bread? I can't eat my pasta? I know that doughnuts are bad for me, but don't take away my pizza!

We've talked about the foods you should be eating to create long and desirable health. Real, live foods should be the basis of any good eating plan. The reason: they reduce systemic inflammation within the body, which has been proven to be the root cause of so many diseases and other issues.

Grains are problematic because they cause inflammation. They contain many anti-nutrients, are nutritionally inferior, are higher in calories, and can be damaging to the gut lining.

WHAT'S IN A GRAIN?

A grain is the seed of a plant or grass and includes barley, oats, corn, rice (including wild rice), rye, wheat (which includes spelt, emmer, farro, kamut, durum, and bulger), millet, teff, triticale, sorghum, amaranth, buckwheat, and quinoa.

ANATOMY OF A GRAIN

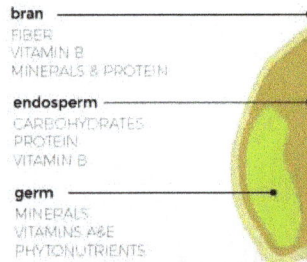

It's comprised of three parts: the bran, the germ, and the endosperm.

bran
FIBER
VITAMIN B
MINERALS & PROTEIN

endosperm
CARBOHYDRATES
PROTEIN
VITAMIN B

germ
MINERALS
VITAMINS A&E
PHYTONUTRIENTS

The bran is the outer layer. It contains antioxidants, B vitamins, and fiber.

The germ is the embryo of the seed. It gives it the potential to sprout into a new plant. It contains some protein, minerals and B vitamins.

The endosperm is the food supply. It provides energy to the plant so that it can grow. It contains starchy carbohydrates, proteins, and small amounts of vitamins and minerals.

Refined grains have both the bran and the germ removed from the seed, so all you're left with is the endosperm. You're missing about 25% of the grain's protein along with the fiber, as well as seventeen key nutrients. Often these nutrients have to be added back to "enrich" refined grains.

What you're essentially left with is an excessively starchy seed, that is often high in gluten, and other gut-irritating anti-nutrients, lacking any natural fibers, and is overall nutritionally imbalanced.

The whole refining process also uses large amounts of chemicals, additives, bleaches, and preservatives to give it a longer shelf life, making it easier to store and transport and ultimately make your flour and bread nice and white.

Refined grains are really nothing more than junk foods that promote overeating, and are high in carbohydrates, which means they ultimately increase body fat, elevate blood sugar levels, and are responsible for a host of related metabolic issues. It's becoming universally agreed upon that refined grains do not make you healthier.

WHAT ABOUT WHOLE GRAINS?

The main difference between refined and whole grains is in the processing. Whole grains contain all three parts of the seed, so they contain all the proteins, natural fiber, vitamins, and minerals that are removed during the refining process. Whole grains are therefore considered a healthier alternative.

We have been inundated with the message that whole grains are "heart healthy" from every government organization that writes our food guides, as well as grain-selling corporations like General Mills (Cheerios, anyone?). We're told they are great sources of dietary fiber, they help reduce cholesterol, and they're low in saturated fats and high in essential vitamins and minerals.

The truth is, they *are* a healthier option...when compared to refined grains. They are still, however, a calorie-dense and nutritionally poor choice when compared to nutrient-dense fruits and vegetables. Here's a chart (see next page) showing some popular nutrient-dense veggies compared to a whole-grain bread.

There is nothing in whole grains that can't be found in fruits and vegetables. Are you worried about fiber? Check out the chart on page 43...veggies win again!

Not to mention that whole grains still contain problematic proteins like gluten and gut-irritating anti-nutrients like lectins and phytic acid.

Common Foods	Serving Size	Fibre (g)
Whole Grain Toast	2 slices	3.8
Oatmeal	1 cup	4
Brown Rice	1 cup	5
Quinoa *	1 cup	3
Pasta	1 cup	3
Broccoli, raw	1.5 cups	3.5
Carrots, raw	1 cup	4
Sweet potato (with skin)	1/2 cup	3.8
Avocado	1/2 avocado	6.5
Apple (medium)	1	4
Raspberries	1 cup	8
Asparagus	1 cup	4
Kale (chopped)	1 cup	5.86

GLUTEN

Gluten is a protein found in wheat, rye, barley, and many other processed foods. It's what gives our favorite foods that special something—it makes our breads spongy and chewy, pizza dough stretchy, and soups and sauces nice and thick.

All wheat contains gluten—including spelt, kamut, bulgur, faro, durum, semolina, barley, triticale and rye. Grains that don't contain gluten are amaranth, buckwheat, corn, millet, oats, quinoa, and rice, although beware of cross-contamination, especially with oats. When you hear the term "gluten free," it typically means free of

Per 100 calories	Wholegrain Bread	Broccoli	Spinach	Tomatoes
Vitamin A (IU)	-	10,714.3	31,428.6	4,627.8
Vitamin C (mg)	0.0	332.9	214.3	70.6
Vitamin B6 (mg)	0.1	0.7	2.1	0.6
Riboflavin (mg)	-	0.4	0.7	-
Calcium (mg)	38.9	171.4	414.3	55.6
Iron (mg)	0.9	3.2	5.7	1.7
Magnesium (mg)	29.4	89.3	278.6	61.1
Phosporous (mg)	86.0	235.7	200.0	133.3
Potassium (mg)	86.8	1,160.7	928.6	1,316.7
Zinc (mg)	0.6	1.4	2.9	1.1

wheat, barley, rye, and their derivatives.

The problem with gluten is that it triggers an autoimmune response that damages the small intestine. You have most likely heard of celiac disease—those who have it cannot eat gluten at all. Eating it sets off a reaction where their immune cells immediately try and destroy the gluten, and in the process attack other cells at the same time. It's now thought that 1 in 133 people have celiac disease, and many more are often misdiagnosed.

The best way to determine sensitivity is to eliminate completely any gluten from your diet for at least thirty days and see if you feel better.

Another issue is gluten sensitivity. This is more prevalent; about thirty to forty percent of Americans are thought to be gluten sensitive. Gluten sensitivity leads to similar symptoms to celiac disease, like stomach cramps, bloating, diarrhea, headaches, joint pain, digestive problems, and weight gain. It creates some type of inflammatory response in your body, can also be damaging to the intestine, and may produce leaky gut. The best way to determine sensitivity is to eliminate completely any gluten from your diet for at least thirty days and see if you feel better.

LECTINS AND PHYTIC ACID

Grains also contain lectins and phytates that cause intestinal damage and immune issues. Lectins are proteins found pretty much everywhere, in all grains and legumes, nuts, and seeds. They bind to your intestinal lining and are associated with leptin resistance. (Leptin's a hormone that regulates your feeling of fullness). Leptin resistance makes you hungrier all the time. They are a major contributor to leaky gut, which leads to autoimmunity and metabolic disease.

Phytates aren't any better. They are anti-nutrients found in gluten and other whole grains and legumes that make minerals bio-unavailable. This means they bind to certain minerals like magnesium, calcium, zinc, and iron and take them out of our bodies, preventing you from absorbing them.

Not what we want. So much for all those healthy vitamins and minerals we're supposed to be getting from whole grains.

LEGUMES: BEANS, BEANS, THEY'RE GOOD FOR... WHAT?

Legumes include all types of beans, peas, lentils, and peanuts. While they are often promoted as an excellent food choice for their vitamins and minerals, fiber, and high protein content, they are not nearly as nutrient or protein dense as other foods like meat, fish, shellfish, eggs, and vegetables. Even their fiber content pales in comparison when compared to vegetables.

One of the main drawbacks of legumes is that they contain a high amount of phytic acid, making them not as nutrient dense as suggested by nutrition data. This may prove especially problematic when they are a large staple food in your diet and are a main source of calories.

They are also high in carbohydrates, which is not necessarily a bad thing, but if you're trying to lose weight, eating a lot of beans and legumes may stall your progress. This in itself is not a reason to stop eating them; however, it's important to mention that taking them out of your diet may help if you're struggling with weight loss.

In addition, legumes are typically harder to digest. They are a type of carbohydrate that is poorly absorbed by most people and can cause a variety of digestive problems, including gas and bloating, and often leads to increased inflammation in your gut.

WHAT ABOUT SOAKING AND SPROUTING?

Soaking, sprouting, and/or fermenting legumes can reduce the lectins and phytates in the foods. These practices have been around for hundreds of years; people knew that if they didn't soak the foods, they would get stomach cramps. If you do choose to eat legumes, soaking and sprouting does make them somewhat healthier, and will make them easier to digest.

SOY

Soy is a hot topic these days. There is a lot of hype surrounding the little bean...is it good or bad? The jury is still out, but one thing's for sure: the benefits of soybeans have been greatly exaggerated, and mostly from a marketing standpoint. It's really not as healthy as it's been presented.

Soy is a **phytoestrogen** (or plant estrogen), meaning it has similar properties to and is recognized by the body as estrogen. Researchers are still out on whether or not it stimulates cancer cells; its effects are unknown. It has, however, been shown to disrupt hormones in both men and women.

If you're going to make soy a part of your regular diet, make sure that it's organic and traditionally fermented soy.

WHERE YOU FIND SOY

PROTEIN BARS
BOTTLED FRUIT DRINKS
BAKED GOODS
BREAKFAST CEREALS
MOST ASIAN FOODS
SOY PROTEIN POWDERS
TOFU
TEMPEH
MISO
SOY SAUCE

Soy is also very new to the food supply—it's only been eaten for about 2000 years. Almost all commercially available soybeans are now genetically modified, and most soy products are overly processed—removing many of its nutritional benefits.

If you're going to make soy a part of your regular diet, make sure that it's organic and traditionally fermented soy.

PEANUTS

Peanuts, despite what you may have thought, are not nuts at all. They are actually considered a legume. They also contain lectins, and while the lectins in other legumes may be destroyed during the cooking process, the lectins in peanuts are not. When you eat them, the proteins are not digested by the body and therefore travel through your gut intact, causing irritation.

Peanuts have a high risk for aflatoxin mold, which make them toxic and potentially carcinogenic. There is also a severe potential for allergic reactions with peanuts.

Instead of peanuts, eat raw tree nuts such as walnuts, almonds, cashews, pecans, or macadamia nuts or their nut butters instead of peanut butter.

TEST IT OUT YOURSELF

Since most of us have been eating grains and legumes all our lives, we may never really know how significantly they affect us until they are removed completely. A little bit of experimentation may go a long way in figuring out just how much or how little they bother you. Eliminating them from your diet for a minimum of thirty days and then re-introducing them is good starting point to see the effects, if any. Only then can you decide for yourself if you want to keep them a part of your diet.

DAIRY: IT DOES A BODY GOOD—OR DOES IT?

We have been so inundated with amazing marketing by the dairy industry that suggests dairy is a miracle food. "You need milk for strong bones" and "Dairy does a body good!" What about the all "Got Milk?" ads from celebrities and athletes, convincing us that we need milk to be healthy? Unless you're breastfeeding (from the same species), dairy, which can refer to milk from cows, sheep, and goats, is not an optimal food choice.

Humans are the only species that drinks another animals' milk and the only one that drinks it past infancy.

MILK PROTEINS

Milk is the most common cause of allergic reactions and intolerance in both children and adults.

This is mainly because of the proteins in dairy, casein and whey—most often casein, which cannot be easily digested by humans. Consuming it can create a huge inflammatory immune response in the body.

IT'S CUSTOM MADE FOR COWS

Humans are the only species that drinks another animals' milk and the only one that drinks it past infancy. Cow milk is an amazing source of nutrients for a calf, just like mother's milk is exceptionally nutritious for her baby. However, **the composition in animal milk is very different from human milk**. For example, cow's milk on average contains three times the amount of protein than human milk does, which can cause huge metabolic disturbances in humans. Calves grow much faster and much bigger than babies do!

EXTREMELY HIGH INSULIN RESPONSE

Milk is a powerful growth promoter, so it only makes sense that it would be highly insulinogenic. This means that the body responds to milk by releasing a large amount of insulin when consumed. When a baby is growing, it needs a lot of insulin to be able to store nutrients—not so much as an adult. Too much insulin will cause hormonal imbalances and metabolic issues, and can stall weight loss. Dairy is actually used to gain mass in bodybuilders.

It can also cause acne and other skin problems, autoimmune issues, mucous buildup, and stuffy noses. Dairy is not ideal if you're looking to improve insulin sensitivity or are insulin resistant.

THE CANCER CONNECTION

We talked about how dairy's purpose is to feed and support the growth of a baby, right? Because of that, milk is full of anabolic hormones, or growth hormones, such as IGF-1. IGF-1 has been pretty consistently linked to promoting growth in certain types of cancer. It's fantastic for growing babies, **not so good for growing cancer cells.**

Milking cows are also often given antibiotics and a bovine growth hormone called rBGH to increase milk production; this also increases IGF-1 levels in those who drink it. It has been shown to increase risks of developing breast cancer and promoting its invasiveness. "Monsanto's Hormonal Milk Poses Serious Risks of Breast Cancer, Besides Other Cancers."

WHAT ABOUT CALCIUM?

The million dollar question! Bone health is super important, but isn't it just a little crazy to think that the only way you can build strong and healthy bones is to eat or drink dairy? Bones need more than just calcium to grow and be strong. There are numerous other vitamins and minerals that contribute, and then there are hormones and your inflammatory status that also play a role.

Many studies have shown that we barely absorb the calcium in cow's milk, especially if it's pasteurized, and that it actually increases calcium loss from bones.

INSTEAD OF DAIRY, TRY THIS FOR CALCIUM:

KALE
BOK CHOY
ALMONDS
SALMON
SARDINES
DRIED FIGS
BROCCOLI
ORANGES
SESAME SEEDS
SEAWEED

It produces acid loads in the body and it forces calcium from the bones in order to neutralize the acid and bring it back to an alkaline state. Hello, osteoporosis. Still think milk does a body good?

LACTOSE INTOLERANCE

Lactose is an issue for alarmingly large number of people—close to 75% of the world's population is lactose intolerant. Lactose is a carbohydrate found in milk that gets converted into the sugars glucose and galactose. If it's not digested properly, symptoms are not fun. They include bloating, gas, diarrhea, cramps as well as itchy skin, eczema, congestion, runny nose and watery eyes.

WHAT ARE THE BEST SUBSTITUTIONS?

Instead of butter, use ghee or clarified butter from grass-fed sources if possible. Ghee is form of butter, but it is free of casein and other milk solids and it's a great source of healthy fats. Coconut milk is another amazing alternative with a lot nutritional value. I've easily transitioned from milk to coconut milk. If you can't find coconut milk, although it's becoming and easier to find, almond milk is the next option. Just make sure that it's unsweetened.

Most of us have been drinking dairy all our lives, so often we really don't know if it affects us negatively or not. I have yet to meet someone, though, who hasn't seen some benefit from removing it from their diet. Again, it's one of those foods that should be experimented with. Take it out of your diet completely for a period of thirty days and see if it has any effect on you. You will never know until you try.

SUGAR: HOW SWEET IT ISN'T

Did you know that the average person is eating about 150 pounds of sugar a year? A hundred years ago we ate about 50 pounds a year, and ten thousand years ago we ate about 25 teaspoons a year. **Sugar is everywhere!** Traditionally, we ate it because our ancestors knew that if a plant was sweet it was okay to eat. (Typically poisonous plants taste bitter). Sweetness also usually meant that the plant was high in glucose, which meant it offered lots of energy.

> Did you know that the average person is eating about 150 pounds of sugar a year? A hundred years ago we ate about 50 pounds a year, and ten thousand years ago we ate about 25 teaspoons a year.

While most people try and avoid the obvious sugar traps like baked goods, sodas, and candy, today it hides in everything, including tomato sauce, fat-free dressings, sports drinks, marinades, and bread. Really, anything processed is bound to have sugar added to it. It's addictive, and manufacturers love that. Sugar sells.

It's totally normal to love sweet things—it's in our genes. At least, it is when we're talking sweetness from natural sources like apples, figs, berries, cherries, and watermelons. When you're eating the whole fruit, including the skin, you're getting all the amazing fiber and nutrients from the food, and the fructose you're consuming is a healthy sugar.

When you take sugar *out* of a plant and add it to

another food, like bread for example, you're not getting any nutritional benefits. It's just added sugar and empty calories.

Eating added or refined sugars puts you on a blood-sugar roller-coaster, with spikes and dips that leave you hungry and then craving more food. It wreaks havoc on your insulin metabolism, raises your stress hormones (making it extremely difficult to burn fat), affects your immune system, helps you store fat, and **has even been shown to feed cancer cells.**

WHERE SUGAR HIDES

If you see any of these words on an ingredient list, it contains sugar!

BARLEY MALT	HONEY
BROWN SUGAR	INVERT SUGAR
CANE JUICE	LACTOSE
CASTOR SUGAR	MALT SUGAR
CORN SWEETENER	MALTODEXTRIN
CORN SYRUP	MALTOSE
CORN SYRUP SOLIDS	MALT
DATE SUGAR	MALT SYRUP
DEXTRIN	MAPLE SYRUP
DEXTROSE	MAPLE SUGAR
EVAPORATED CANE JUICE	MOLASSES
FRUCTOSE	RAW SUGAR
FRUIT JUICE CONCENTRATE	RICE SYRUP
GALACTOSE	SUCROSE (TABLE SUGAR)
GLUCOSE	TREACLE
HIGH-FRUCTOSE CORN SYRUP (HFCS)	TURBINADO

When you think about sugar, the first things that come to mind are candies, cakes, and all things tasty-sweet. But in reality, all carbohydrates, both complex (the good ones, unrefined) and simple (the bad ones, refined and processed), are broken down into glucose in the body. Glucose is the main source of fuel for your brain, and you want a steady supply of it.

A LITTLE ON GLUCOSE...

Once glucose hits your bloodstream, the pancreas releases a hormone called insulin. Insulin lowers the level of glucose in the blood by helping it enter into the cells so the cell has fuel to provide you energy. Once that cell has all the fuel it needs, insulin takes the rest of the glucose away to store it as fat.

A diet high in simple and refined sugars dumps a lot of glucose into your system, and very quickly—which means your pancreas releases a lot more insulin to try and shuttle it into your cells, but the sugar cannot get in. When this happens, you become insulin-resistant. This not only makes losing weight extremely difficult, but too much glucose and insulin is a major cause of metabolic syndrome, Type 2 diabetes, and a host of other diseases.

A LITTLE ON SUGAR AND CANCER...

It has been well documented in literature that there is in fact a link between insulin resistance and cancer. Cancer cells are extremely hungry, and their preferred fuel is glucose. Excess insulin tells cancer cells to grow.

Controlling your blood-sugar levels through diet, supplements, exercise, and mediation can be a huge

The explanation is a little complex. There is a lot of documented work by Nobel laureate in medicine Dr. Otto Warburg, who first discovered that cancer cells metabolize energy differently than healthy cells. All normal cells meet their energy needs by respiration (the process by which nutrients are converted to energy) of oxygen; cancer cells meet their energy needs in large part through fermentation, which converts sugar to energy without using oxygen. **So the best way to feed cancer cells is to keep eating lots of simple carbs and lots of sugar.**

Have you ever heard of a PET scan? It's a test where they inject you with radioactive glucose and measure where the body absorbs most of the sugar. Cancer cells light up like fireflies.

That's all I needed to know when I was diagnosed with cancer. I really wasn't going to take the chance. Beginning during my treatments and continuing to this day, I do a ketogenic diet for six to eight weeks once or twice a year. Remember how I told you that our bodies don't actually need carbohydrates to survive? A ketogenic diet removes the majority of carbs from your diet, and your body is fueled by fat instead.

Removing sugar from your diet is essential for optimal health.

SO HOW DO I MAKE BETTER CHOICES WHEN IT COMES TO SUGAR?

Use the glycemic index.

The glycemic index is a rating system developed to

measure how the foods you eat affect your blood sugar levels. Glucose is set at 100, and all other carbs will vary. Carbs that break down quickly and release sugar fast are rated higher than ones that break down slowly and release sugar more gradually. Foods that are lower are generally less refined and have more fiber, whereas foods that have a higher value are almost always refined, simple carbs. Get familiar with it, it's a great tool.

Keep in mind that the glycemic index doesn't take into account the amount of food eaten in a serving. It also doesn't decipher between good and poor nutritional choices. A watermelon is rated high, at 72, whereas a snickers bar comes up lower at 32. Which one do you think is the healthier option?

HOW DO YOU CURB SUGAR CRAVINGS?

- **Eat more protein.**
  Eating the right amount of protein three to four times a day can work wonders on your blood-sugar levels. Not enough protein can contribute to sugar cravings, as the body will look for a quick energy source.

- **Toss the artificial sweeteners.**
  The taste of sugar, real or fake, has the same effect on the body and creates cravings for more. Not only that, but artificial sweeteners of any kind—aspartame, Splenda, Equal, Sweet 'n Low, saccharin, etc.—are potent nerve toxins that should never have been allowed for human consumption. They damage your nervous system and have even been linked to cancer.

- **Spice it up.**
  Learn to use spices like coriander, cinnamon, nutmeg, cloves,

and cardamom, which will naturally add sweetness, so you don't need the sugar.

- **Retrain your taste buds.**
  If you're used to eating a lot of sugary things, you've most definitely overstimulated your tastebuds. Let mother nature remind you how sweet natural and real foods actually are. You will be surprised!

IF YOU HAVE A SWEET TOOTH...

- **Have some chocolate.**
  Make sure it's dark chocolate—75% cacao or higher—and make sure it's a small piece.

- **Eat an apple with almond butter and sprinkled with cinnamon.**

- **Roast a sweet potato and add some cinnamon.**

- **Mix some cacao powder into coconut milk and add some berries on top.**

- **Snack on low-glycemic fruits, like berries or pears.**

- **Move!**
  Go for a walk, call a friend, get your nails done. A craving won't last for more than twenty minutes. Distract yourself until it passes.

> Sugar is not a nutrient, and you don't need it as a part of a healthy diet. Ditch the processed stuff, read your labels, and avoid added sugars.

Remember that all sugars are not created equal. There are many different kinds. Over the last hundred years we've fallen hard for them, and we're now starting to pay the price. Sugar is not a nutrient, and you don't need it as a part of a healthy diet. Ditch the processed stuff, read your labels, and avoid added sugars. Do allow yourself to share a dessert with your friends every once in while, but not on a daily basis—make fruit your go-to treat instead.

1.7 WATER: ARE YOU DRINKING ENOUGH?

Water is the most abundant and important substance both on Earth and in the human body. Three simple molecules—two hydrogen and one oxygen—and it makes up 70% of your body. It's responsible for pretty much every function of your body, from circulation, digestion, and absorption, to elimination. It's the main component of blood and lymph, and it's responsible for every chemical reaction in the body.

It's absolutely essential for optimal health.

It's amazingly healing, both physically and psychologically. When we're injured, our bloodstream brings the wound substances to repair it—and our bloodstream is 80% water. When toxins enter our bodies, we most often get rid of them through sweat and urine— both comprised of 95% water. Hot tubs, baths, a swim, even the mere sight of a lake, ocean, or waterfall can be extremely healing. And water is essential for weight loss. It will help you get healthy and lose weight faster than any other substance.

You can probably live for about a month without food, but wouldn't last a week if you didn't have any access to water.

Water is fundamental to life, and without clean water we can't experience optimal health. You need it to survive. You can probably live for about a month without food, but wouldn't last a week if you didn't have any access to water. And without enough of it, we basically dry up, or become dehydrated. Many people experience dehydration without even realizing it. Fatigue, headaches, loss of appetite, feeling really hot or lightheaded and nauseous are all symptoms of dehydration.

Water is fundamental to life, and without clean water we can't experience optimal health. You need it to survive.

Are you thirsty? Unfortunately, we haven't been given a very good thirst monitor. **By the time you're thirsty, you're probably already dehydrated.**

Check your pee! Is it pale or dark? Dark urine is a sure sign you should be drinking more water. Urine that's pale yellow indicates you are within 1% of optimal hydration.

STAYING HYDRATED

On average, we should be consuming about half of our body weight in ounces of water each day.

That means for a 130 pound woman, she would need about two liters (nine cups) of total fluids a day. This, of course, is just a baseline. If you're exercising, spending a lot of time in hot or dry weather, or drinking a lot of caffeinated drinks (which pull water and minerals from your body—think coffee, teas or soda), you're going to need more water.

Also keep in mind that you shouldn't drink water with or just after meals as it can dilute digestive juices and reduce food digestion, so you may not be assimilating your nutrients as effectively as possible.

AMP UP THE FLAVOUR OF YOUR WATER

- **Add a handful of frozen berries to your water bottle.**
  It will keep your water cool and add amazing flavour

- **Add some lemon, lime, oranges, or all three.**
  You get a tasty drink plus the added nutrients.

- **Make natural herbal teas instead of water.**
  You can drink them hot or add ice!

- **Eat your fruits and veggies.**
  Fruit is typically more than 90% water, so when you're eating that juicy peach or tasty watermelon, you're absorbing all the water they hold.

CAN YOU DRINK TOO MUCH WATER?

It's very rare, but it can happen. Drinking too much can lead to a condition called water intoxication, or hyponatremia, which happens when you dilute the electrolytes in your body. It's most often seen in athletes who consume a lot of water and lose a lot of salt through sweat. Nine cups of water per day will not over-hydrate your body.

GRAB A FILTER, DITCH THE BOTTLE

Not all water is created equal, and since it's the substance we need the most, we should know what the water we drink contains. According to Health Canada, our drinking water is generally of excellent quality. However, it's never pure. Water likes to move down from mountaintop snow to lowland watersheds and farther down through soil and rock and then becomes groundwater. Along the way it picks up multiple minerals, like calcium and magnesium, making it very supportive to our health. It also picks up many of the toxins that have found their way into the soil and groundwater. Everything from fertilizers, pesticides, sewage, waste contaminants, and toxins released into the air by manufacturing companies all contribute to the toxicity of our water.

A CBC article titled "Is our water safe to drink" reported that on any given day there are an estimated 1,500 boil water advisories in effect across Canada. Some are in effect for hours, some for days—and some have lasted decades." For the most part, **city water is heavily chlorinated to kill germs and has a lot fluoride in it** to prevent tooth decay; some cities even add chemicals to the water to change the pH (acidity) of the water so it doesn't corrode the pipes.

What to do? Use purified water and avoid the faucet. Request a water report from your municipality and have your tap water tested for bacterial count, mineral content, and the presence of any chemicals. If there's a concern, add a filtration system or a purification system to your home. At a minimum, put a filter on your kitchen tap for your drinking water, but remember that your skin is your biggest organ and absorbs substances just as though you were drinking them.

Consider installing a system for your whole house. In the long run they are the least expensive and safest way to get safe, good-tasting water.

THE MOST COMMON SYSTEMS:

- **Activated Carbon.**
Activated carbon chemically attaches and removes contaminants in water that is filtered through it. It can remove unpleasant appearance, odor, and taste by cleaning the water of bacteria, parasites, most viruses, chlorine, and heavier minerals and matter. It's not so good as removing inorganic materials like fluoride or heavy metals like lead or mercury.

- **Reverse Osmosis.**
Some believe reverse osmosis (RO) is the best way to purify water. This process pushes water through a really small filter that blocks particles larger than water molecules. It can remove a lot of the contaminants not removed by activated carbon, including fluoride. However, RO does not remove chlorine or VOCs (like solvent residues). Pretty much all organic material is removed along with the minerals. They are not very water efficient. They use three to twenty times more water than they produce. Because of this they are best used for drinking and cooking water only.

- **Pitcher filters.**
While you're researching the best home filtration system for

you, the simplest and cheapest way to treat drinking water is to buy a pitcher that has a built-in filter, like a Brita or a Soma water carafe and filter. It's a glass pitcher with the first fully biodegradable filter made from coconut shells. Pretty awesome!

DITCH THE BOTTLE

Yes, its so easy to go pick up a bottle of water, but what are you really buying? Is it pure, clean and fresh from pools of spring water or high mountain peaks? Not likely.

In reality, bottled water is just water. Most of it comes from your municipal supply. It's treated, purified, and then sold to us for at an insanely increased cost in price.

Are you surprised? Visit Dasani's website, where they acknowledge their supply is from local water. Aquafina states on their label its water comes from public water sources. Why do we keep buying glorified tap water that really isn't any healthier than the water from your kitchen tap? It's costly and it's wasteful and the plastic can be dangerous to your health.

Bottled water also means a lot of garbage. It

At a minimum, put a filter on your kitchen tap for your drinking water, but remember that your skin is your biggest organ and absorbs substances just as though you were drinking them.

produces up 1.5 million tons of plastic garbage a year, and although some of it is recycled, according to Food and Water Watch, over 80% of plastic bottles are just thrown away.

The plastic bottles themselves may contain chemicals called BPAs, which can affect your hormones. Not a risk I'm willing to take. A quick and simple alternative to bottled water is buying a reusable stainless steel bottle like Kleen Kanteen—or even a glass bottle will do. Stay away from the plastics!

Bottoms up!

PART 2 :: FITNESS - LET'S MOVE! THE BASICS OF BUILDING A STRONG BODY

2.1 YOUR BODY WANTS TO BE STRONG!

It's your birthright! Don't ever think that you were meant to be anything but. Your body wants to be powerful and resilient. It wants to be beautiful and strong. It wants to be exactly the way you envision it! We, by nature, are programmed for survival, so it's only natural for our bodies to be strong and healthy—that way we are able to create more strong and capable bodies. Our survival depends on it.

Back in the day, our ancestors didn't stop moving from morning to night. They built strong bodies out of necessity. They didn't have the luxuries of modern technology that we do. They had to physically go out and hunt and forage for food, they had to build shelters, move heavy loads without machines—all things that required strength and movement on a daily basis each and every day.

Let's not even go that far. As early as a hundred years ago, people still had to wash and dry their own clothes, care for livestock, maintain wagons, fix their own homes, dig in the dirt, get water from the well or nearest stream. We didn't have cars, kids ran and played outside, and they had to actually walk to school! We were physically active all day long.

Today we wake up, drive to the office, sit all day long at a desk, grab our food from the nearest drive-thru, drive home from work, and to relax and unwind, we sit in front of the TV for the rest of the night. Our lifestyles have become so sedentary and devoid of movement–is it really a surprise that we are getting weaker? **We have become a society that loves to sit!** With modern-day conveniences, we can pretty much do everything we need to do, from grocery shopping to socializing with friends through social media from the couch!

A weak body is the perfect host and nesting ground for illness. Instead of building bodies that are strong enough to fight off modern-day lions like disease, we are weakening our bodies through lack of proper nutrition and movement.

When we are not careful about what we eat and how move we become prone to illness. Type 2 diabetes, heart disease, autoimmune diseases, and even cancer have become the norm. Obesity is skyrocketing, and our immune systems are too weak to cope.

You were meant to move all day long and rest and repair for eight hours a day, not twenty-four!

Moving your body throughout the day is essential to creating a strong and healthy life. You were meant to move all day long and rest and repair for eight hours a day, not twenty-four!

2.2 BUILDING HEALTHY BONES

Bones are truly the support system of the body. Strong, yet light, they have perfectly adapted for their functions of protecting the body and movement! They form the internal framework of our bodies, they protect our soft organs, and allow the body to move. Our bones are also a storehouse for minerals, and they're where blood-cell formation happens. Although the word *skeleton* comes from the Greek word meaning "dried-up body," our bones are far from that. They are living tissues, and they grow and change throughout our lifetime.

Bones are constantly being broken down and re-built. The majority of growth happens up until about our twenties, with peak bone mass being reached at about thirty. After that, more bone is lost than gained, and our bones turn into re-building mode instead of growth mode. It's why you won't see most people grow taller past their teenage years, and it's also why it's particularly important to build a good foundation of strong and healthy bones in kids and teens. Moms and dads of kids, take note! In order for new growth to happen, nutrients need to be available and things that weaken bones need to be minimized. Just as importantly, bones need exercise to stay strong and healthy.

As we age and especially in our early to mid forties, we start to lose more bone than we create. How much is lost varies from person to person. Some lose more than others and it is often dependent on age, genetics, hormones, and how much bone mass you've built up as a kid. Once your bones start to lose more than they can build, they become brittle and weak. Hello, osteoporosis! You're now on your way to getting fractured more easily. With weaker bones, a little slip can cause serious breaks!

YOUR ACTION PLAN

Granted, there are some things that you're not going to be able to change. If you're twenty-five or younger and reading this...get on it now and build, build, build! Bones get stronger when you use them. If you're forty, you can't turn back the clock but there are things you can do minimize your bone loss and bump up your bone density starting today.

Exercise!! Working out builds bones, period. Being sedentary decreases bone density, and has even been labeled as a risk factor for osteoporosis, just like smoking and a bad diet. Movement and exercise are essential.

The most effective exercises are those that involve weight or some type of resistance against gravity. Muscle contraction signals the body to put minerals into the bones, especially the hips, spine, and legs. Any exercise that places force on the bone will strengthen it.

On the other hand, there are exercises that may decrease bone density. Exercises like swimming and biking are two, because your body is supported either by the bike or the water and there is no force or resistance placed on your bones.

Add the following exercises to your training routine as much and as often as possible:

• **Weightlifting**....yes, with weight! Start light and work your way up!

  • **Any bodyweight exercise**

  • **Squats**

  • **Lunges**

  • **Gymnastics**

  • **Pull-ups**

  • **Push-ups**

  • **Jumping rope**

  • **Plyometrics**

  • **Running/jogging**

  • **Stairs**

  • **Sprints**

  • **Walking**

- Skipping

- Dancing

- Yoga

Building strong bones is something you have to work at—it won't happen on its own, and it's never too late to start.

2.3 GETTING TO KNOW YOUR BODY

Ladies, your **strength is sexy...muscles included!**

Like most women, my main motivation at first for getting a gym membership was purely aesthetic. I had a very poor body image as a teenager and in my early twenties. I struggled with how I looked, I had a huge issue with my "big" thighs and butt, and after giving birth to the twins and my youngest baby girl, I was itching to get into shape—and, more importantly, into my jeans.

Very quickly, though, my love for strength training developed into something I had never imagined. Lifting weights became less about how I looked and more about how I felt. **It was empowering to see what I was capable of. It taught me that I can create my own strength.** I began to believe in my own abilities. Strength training builds confidence physically, emotionally, and mentally. Lifting weights and reaching new goals gives you a sense of personal pride. Lifting weights and reach-

> Strength training builds confidence physically, emotionally, and mentally.

ing new goals gives you a sense of personal pride. I could easily carry my kids, carry all the groceries, chop wood, move the furniture all on my own, and eventually battle cancer too.

During my cancer treatments, getting to the gym and training was both a mental and a physical push. Even though my body was beaten and broken, training made me feel strong. I could feel my body growing and healing with every sweaty session. I would leave the gym more energized than ever.

The best part was that for the first time ever, I really felt connected to my body. I felt my muscles working, I began to understand what they did and how important it was to be strong. Aside from all the health benefits, lifting weights gave me an awareness of how truly powerful the body is.

I was intrigued by my body. I wanted to learn more about all the good aches and pains I was feeling after every workout, and which remarkable muscles were responsible. We have about 642 skeletal muscles, and they all help our bodies move.

UPPER-BODY MUSCLES

- ### Trapezius
  The trapezius muscle is a diamond-shaped muscle located on the upper back, neck, and shoulders. Its main function is to move the scapulae, or shoulder blades, and support the arms. It's a fairly large muscle and most visible in athletes around the neck area. Explosive lifting is the secret to well-developed traps. Olympic lifting are some of the best movements. If you want to build strong traps, clean and jerks and snatches are the way to go!

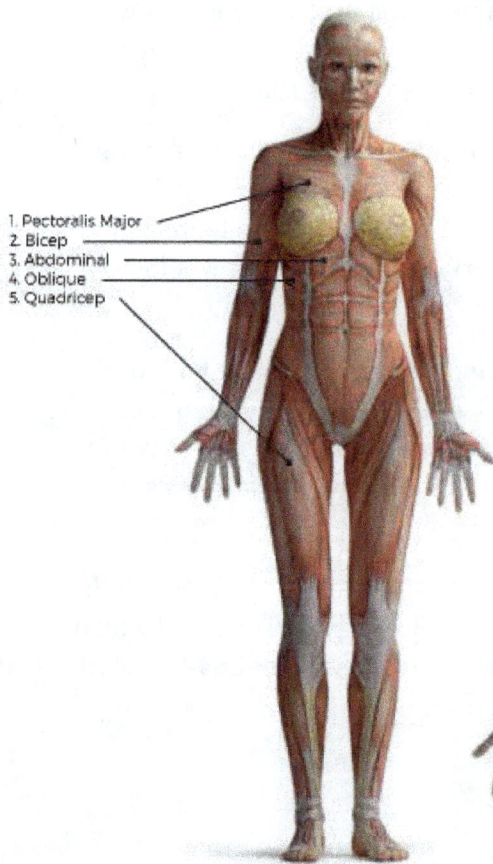

1. Pectoralis Major
2. Bicep
3. Abdominal
4. Oblique
5. Quadricep

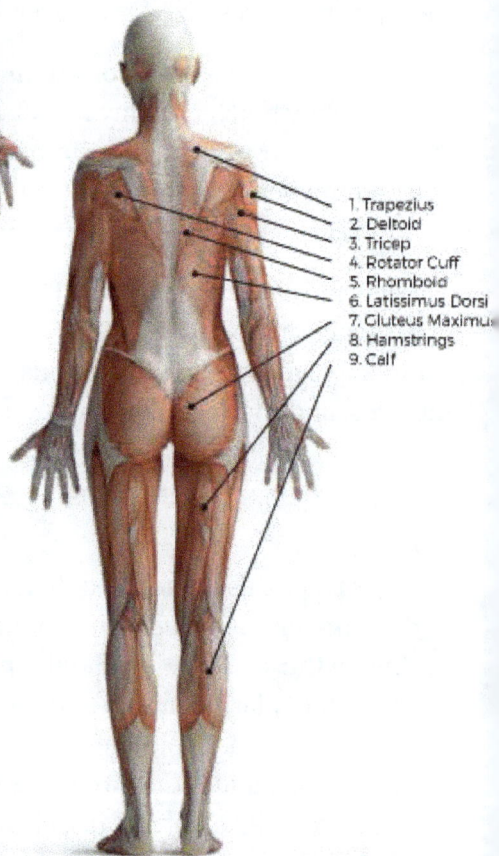

1. Trapezius
2. Deltoid
3. Tricep
4. Rotator Cuff
5. Rhomboid
6. Latissimus Dorsi
7. Gluteus Maximus
8. Hamstrings
9. Calf

- **Deltoid**

  The deltoids are triangular-shaped muscles that form the rounded shape of your shoulders. They are responsible for any side lifting movements as well as any movement of your upper arms and scapulae. Pretty much all movements above the elbow joint. Your deltoids are responsible for any pushing and pulling movements to the front of the body or above the head like pushups, bench presses, or shoulder presses. They are also responsible for pulling exercises, such as pull-ups and rows and any movements that move the arms away from the body.

- **Rhomboid**

  The rhomboids are located in the upper back under your traps and are responsible for pulling your shoulder blades together and also rotating the scapulae downward to provide stability for the shoulder complex. They are particularly important in stabilizing any overheard lifts like snatches or overhead squats. How's your posture? Shoulders that are rounded forward, like the Hunchback of Notre Dame, may be a sign of weakened rhomboids.

- **Chest**

  This is a muscle group that guys spend hours on end in the gym working on and most often left out by women. A "firmer chest" isn't usually on the wish list of ladies when they start the gym, but a well-rounded program should definitely include chest training. Ladies, it won't make your boobs smaller–or firmer, for that matter. It *will* strengthen the muscles under the fat that makes up your breasts. Adding muscle will help you appear fuller!

The chest is made up of two muscles: the *pectoralis major* and the *pectoralis minor*. The pectoralis major makes up the majority of the chest muscle you see in males. In females it lies underneath the breast. The pectoralis major brings the arms across the body, while the pectoralis minor, which sits under the pectoralis major, moves the shoulders forward. You use it lifting a child or throwing a ball. There are many exercises that work the pectoral muscles. Include in your routine the bench press, overhead press, weighted dips, and pushups.

- **Back**

    The *latissimus dorsi* muscles, often referred to as lats, are the largest muscles of the back and sit on either side of the back-bone and cover the lower back. They are a very powerful muscle and mainly responsible for the movement of the shoulders. They are also very important when the arm must be brought down in a power stroke, as when swimming or punching.

The *erector spinae* are a group of muscles that are the prime movers of back extension. They are deep muscles of the back and span its entire length. Back extensors help you bend forward at the waist and back and laterally as well.

Strong back muscles make everyday activities easier, and they help you look great in a backless dress!

Lats are the main muscle used when doing both wide-grip and close-grip pull-ups. Other great exercises are barbell rows and deadlifts for your spinal erectors and the lower back.

ARM MUSCLES

• Bicep

The bicep is the most familiar muscle of the arm, because it bulges when the elbow is flexed. Flex your arm and squeeze and there it is! The biceps are responsible for pulling movements, like rows and pull-ups. They help to bring your arm closer to your body and they help to rotate the forearm. The best way to remember it is to think of opening a bottle of wine. Turn the corkscrew, and then flex the elbow to pull the cork.

• Tricep

The triceps are a major muscle of the upper arm. They run along the main bone of the upper arm between the shoulder and the elbow. The triceps are the muscles opposite the biceps, and they are responsible for extension of the elbow, or straightening of the arm. They are also, along with the lats, responsible for bringing the arm closer to the body.

This muscle is sometimes called the "boxer's" muscle, because it can deliver a straight-arm knockout punch. Great exercises for stronger triceps are close-grip bench press and dips (weighted).

CORE MUSCLES

• Abdominals

The abdominals, or abs, are a group of muscles located in the midsection of the body. Most people train them because they want that six-pack for the summer, but the real job of your abdominals has nothing to do with looking good. They support the upper and lower body, provide movement and postural support, help with breathing, and are a key component to athletic ability.

Most sports and really everyday activities have some twisting or rotation—think golf swings or turning to catch a ball. The abs work with the back muscles to control the motion. Moving your upper and lower body at the same time would be extremely difficult without a strong core. Swimming, rowing, throwing—all need coordination and control, and strong abs help to connect these movements and support midline stabilization. When you breathe, your abs contract and push the diaphragm up, forcing air out of the lungs. Better breathing can increase performance, endurance and recovery.

Any exercises that help to stabilize the midsection will develop amazing core strength.

Squats, deadlifts, and overhead presses are great exercises for developing the core, as are Turkish getups, farmer's walks, plank variations, and even sprinting. A thousand sit-ups a day alone will not get you there! Running, jumping, punching, and throwing all come from the core.

If you're looking for those washboard abs, the key is to build a strong core and eat well. Once you build the foundation and dial in your diet, you'll start to see all that hard-earned muscle.

LOWER-BODY MUSCLES

MUSCLES CAUSING HIP JOINT MOVEMENT—HIPS

- **Gluteus**
Ah, the *gluteus maximus*, or the beautiful buttock. It's made up

of three muscles that sit on the hip bone: the gluteus maximus, medius, and minimus. The gluteus maximus is one of the strongest muscles in the body, and it's primarily responsible for bringing your thigh in a straight line with your pelvis. It forms the bulk of your butt and it is probably the most important muscle when power is needed, as in climbing stairs or jumping. The gluteus medius and minimus help to steady you when walking or running.

The path to a better booty is found under a barbell, ladies. You have to target the butt from many angles to engage all muscles involved, and there are many ways to do this. The best exercise is the tried and tested squat. You must squat, squat some more, and then, yes, squat some more! Deadlifts, plyometrics, and any single-leg exercises like walking lunges, overhead lunges, stepups, and pistols are great tools, too, for building that sexy derriere!

MUSCLES CAUSING MOVEMENT AT THE KNEE JOINT—THIGH

• **Hamstrings**
The muscles that form the back of your thigh are called the hamstrings and are made up of three different muscle groups. They cross two joints, the hip and knee and are therefore mainly responsible for flexing or bending the knee and extending the hip (moving the upper leg backwards). The hamstrings play a major role in in transferring power between the hip and knee during athletic movement. If your hamstrings lack strength and flexibility, you won't be able to run as fast or jump as far.

For those that spend most of their day sitting, the hamstrings are often shortened and weak. Improving hamstring strength will increase knee stability and decrease your risk of knee pain and injury. Train the squat, deadlift, and include Olympic lifts. Romanian deadlifts, good mornings, and glute-ham raises are great exercises to build strength–and don't forget to stretch!

- **Quadriceps**

  The quads are a group of four muscles found at the front of the thigh. Their function is to extend the knee, straightening the leg, and to flex the hip. The quads are the largest and most powerful muscle group in the body, which make sense because they have to move the biggest bone, your femur. Grab your ankle and pull it back towards your butt and push your hips forward. Do you feel that stretch in upper front part of your leg? Those are your quadriceps.

It's also important to know that all four muscles attach to your knee and play a huge role in stabilizing it. Strength work on the quads can make a big difference in keeping your knees aligned and stable.

To engage your thighs, stand up with your back against the wall and slowly bend down to a sitting position. Hold that for thirty seconds and release.

MUSCLES CAUSING MOVEMENT AT THE ANKLE AND FOOT—LEG

- **Calf**

  The calf is made up two muscles known as the *gastrocnemius* and *soleus* muscles and is responsible for bending the foot back at the ankle, bending the knee, and helping to move and stabilize when you walk run or jump. Stand on your toes and hold it for 5-6 seconds–now you're working your calves. Jumping rope, farmer's walk on your toes, Olympic lifting, and pushing a sled are great ways to strengthen and build your calf muscles.

2.4 BUILDING A STRONG FOUNDATION

The basis of any great program design is strength. You must build a strong foundation first!

Building a strong body begins with building a strong structure—just like when you're building a house, you first need to pour concrete for the base; or when you're building a car, you need the chassis. When you want to build a strong body, your bones and muscles are that foundation, and however strong that foundation is will determine how long that structure will hold you up throughout your life.

Now, don't get all freaked out about this! If you're envisioning crazy amounts of weight sitting on your back, huge body-builders...stop. Your choice of weight is determined by what you can do right now,

> The basis of any great program design is strength. You must build a strong foundation first!

but remember you can't build muscle using five-pound dumb-bells. Your purse weighs more than that! It doesn't have to be crazy heavy at the start, there just has to be resistance.

HERE'S WHY:

- **Strength training or weight training is one of the most effective ways to burn fat and build muscle.**
It's a great way to increase your metabolic rate. Some studies have shown that it can boost your metabolism for up to for-ty-eight hours after your workout as your body pays off oxygen debt, replenishes its energy reserves, and repairs muscle tis-sue. It also helps by speeding up your Resting Metabolic Rate (RMR). This is because it takes more calories to maintain mus-cle than it does to maintain fat. Regular strength training will raise your RMR in as little as three months. Adding two pounds of muscle burns an extra 65 calories a day; that's 2015 calories per month, and equal to losing half a pound of fat!

- **It makes you healthier.**
Strength training increases bone density, and can prevent os-teoporosis and muscle and bone loss, which all helps us to stay independent, age more gracefully, and stay alive and vibrant and out of a nursing home. Those who strength train have stronger immune systems. It builds a stronger heart, improves blood flow, helps control blood sugar, improves cholesterol lev-els, reduces cancer risk, and improves your posture, balance, and coordination.

- **It makes you feel great.**
Nothing is more satisfying than the feeling of a great workout. I bet you've never heard anyone say, "I wish I didn't work out

today, now I feel like crap!" Lifting weights will give you more energy and confidence. You'll feel less stress and anxiety and you'll continue your day in a better overall mood, because moving is essential for a healthy brain.

- **You'll look great naked!**
For many, this is one of the main benefits of strength training. After all, most people start training just for this purpose alone—getting a fit and toned body. Nothing wrong with that. We all want to look fantastic, don't we!

- **You'll sleep better.**
Exercise can help you sleep more soundly at night. It has been shown to improve insomnia.

- **Your health will improve.**
Strength training has also been proven to help manage and improve the quality of life for people with arthritis, Parkinson's Disease, lymphedema, fibromyalgia, cancer, clinical depression... the list goes on and on. I couldn't find one study that showed strength training had a negative effect on anyone. It's beneficial for everyone from kids to your eighty-year-old grandmother. You're never to old or too young to start!

You have a lifetime to spend in that body you have, make it a strong one!

You have a lifetime to spend in that body you have, make it a strong one!

So how do you do build that body? Building strength and muscle is a choice that you make everyday with the foods you eat and the activities that you do. Nourishing your body, training functional movements, and maximizing the development of the ten fitness abilities—strength, power, endurance, speed, mobility, agility, coordination, stability, balance, and flexibility—should be your focus to get the best results.

LIFT WEIGHTS

Yes, yes, you must! You are not going to be able to see or make any changes by just thinking about it. **You must move, sweat, dig deep, and lift some weight to get results.** Don't worry, it's not going to turn you into the female version of Arnold Schwarzenegger. It will turn you into one sexy lady, though, both inside and out!

If you've never trained before, please be kind to yourself. Understand that major changes do not happen overnight—but progress does. It's taken you years to develop the body you have right now at this moment. It will take some time to make changes. Don't be discouraged and stay consistent. Most athletes take years to develop their bodies and their abilities when it comes to their sport. Lots and lots of dedication, sacrifice, patience, passion, and drive is at the heart of all their success.

You can start sweating today, right now, and start to see progress, but it's important to set yourself up for success. Don't compare yourself and your abilities to others. The only person you should be competing with is yourself! Every day, push to be better than yesterday. Learn about your body and its movements. **Make sure you're always training with proper form.**

Find a sport or activity that challenges you and keeps you coming back for more. Prepare to make this a lifetime commitment. You have to build that body! You can do it!!

HERE'S HOW:

Train functional movements. Functional movements are movements that you do naturally every day. Running, walking, squatting, lunging, pushing, pulling, rotation, throwing, jumping, and lifting things above your head are all things our bodies are meant to do—it's in our DNA.

Functional exercises often involve multi-joint and multi-muscle exercises. They use compound movements, meaning they use several muscle groups to move two or more joints through a range of motion. For example, the squat uses the ankles, knees, and hips, and stresses the quads, hamstrings, glutes, back, and core, and a whole bunch of other stabilizing muscles. It works many parts of the body at the same time. Isolation movements, such as a bicep curl, target only a single joint—the elbow. Train compound movements often. They build muscle fast and strengthen the body as a whole. And they build athleticism.

Training compound movements also elicits a high neuroendocrine response, which results in a higher hormonal response in the body. More testosterone and more human growth hormone means faster strength building. It's like a natural steroid! Who needs drugs when you can squat and deadlift?

WHICH COMPOUND EXERCISES ARE BEST?

This type of training, if properly executed, can make everyday activities easier. If you train the muscles to work the way they do every day, you will prepare your body to be able to perform well in any situation. Here's how you can incorporate functional movements into your training.

EXERCISE NAME	MAJOR MUSCLE GROUPS	MINOR MUSCLE GROUPS
Squats	Quads, hamstrings, glutes, lower back	Lower legs, upper back, core stabilizing muscles, hip complex
Deadlift	Grip, lower back, hamstrings, traps, back of shoulders	Lower legs, core, upper legs, isometric work for biceps, & virtually everything else
Bench Press	Pecs, triceps, front of shoulders	Serratus muscles at side of ribs, side of shoulders, neck
Pullups (rows)	Lats & upper back, biceps, grip	Core, neck
Overhead pressing	Shoulders, triceps	Core stabilizing muscles, neck

BODYWEIGHT AND GYMNASTICS MOVEMENTS

A simple and effective way to get moving without any equipment. You can do bodyweight exercises anywhere–at the gym, on vacation in your hotel room, in the park, on your lunch break, or on your living room floor, using your own body's weight as resistance.

The nice thing about these exercises is that they are very safe and natural and can be done by most people. Bodyweight exercises are a must for any great training program. Once you've mastered the basics of bodyweight exercises, add some tools for greater gains. Grab a pull-up bar, some gymnastics rings, and a climbing rope–if you're just beginning, grab an exercise band to help you.

Work on squats, pull-ups, pushups, dips, sit-ups, running, lunging, sprinting, handstands, splits, roll overs, climbing ropes and walls, and jumping rope!

DUMBBELLS

Dumbbells are a great next step and way to add resistance to your training. One of their advantages is convenience. **You can do dumbbell exercises anywhere from the gym to your living room floor.** Heck, every gym usually has a set tucked away in the corner, usually collecting dust. Check them out the next time you're on vacation! They are easy to find and a fairly inexpensive way to work out your entire body. If you want grab a set and keep them at home, they take up little space and cost far less than many other types of equipment.

Dumbbells are a great way to train all your muscle groups, from top to bottom. They allow for full range of motion when working various areas of the muscle, and the instability will force both sides of the body to work independently.

The one disadvantage to dumbbells is that you may outgrow the weight. As you improve your strength, you'll need to move up in weight to continue gaining strength.

You can use dumbbells to do anything from deadlifts to running. The possibilities are endless. Get some!

BARBELLS

Woot, woot, my favourite! Barbells make you stronger, leaner, and more athletically muscular than any other form of exercise. If you want to improve absolute, maximum strength, you need to use barbells. Build muscle? Barbells! Lose weight? Barbells!

Barbells make you stronger, leaner, and more athletically muscular than any other form of exercise.

Barbells train strength, power, endurance, coordination, speed, and accuracy, to name a few. It incorporates the core muscles, which lead to strong stabilizer muscles—six-pack, anyone? They use big muscle groups, which allows you to move heavy weights that require full body strength and huge energy expenditure. There is no exercise that can replace a heavy barbell squat and deadlift. It helps to build strength and improves physical ability that can be used in the real world, every day!

Barbell training will not make you big and bulky, ladies...more on that later. It's quite the opposite. There is no other piece of equipment that has the same amazing benefits as training with a barbell. It doesn't have to be exclusive, but it should be an important part of everyone's training program.

The bottom line is, you need to lift heavy things that involve compound movements! Nothing will have a more dramatic and positive effect on your body.

NEXT...

Train each workout explosively. Working the Olympic lifts, like the clean, snatch and jerk can improve overall strength immensely, increase metabolism, and improve your fitness. Regardless of weight, there is huge benefit in moving loads as fast as possible. It develops fast twitch muscle fibers, so it helps to develop strength and power.

FOCUS ON FORM

Before you start lifting any kind of weight, you have make sure your form is correct. This I can't stress enough. **Form is everything!** You must use your body's mechanics the right way in order to get the most out every movement. It is just as important to a beginner to master good form as it is to an experienced athlete who is lifting that weight for the millionth time.

Bad form means your body is not moving efficiently and will inevitably lead to injury. Make sure you learn proper form from a reliable source right from the start. Don't be afraid to ask, and make sure that anyone who is coaching you knows that form is important to you and that you welcome their feedback and want them to correct you until you get it right.

> "It's not what you are that holds you back, it's what you think you are not."
>
> *Denis Waitley*

WILL I GET BULKY?

You will NOT get bulky from lifting heavy things.

Let's face it, building a strong body is usually not the first reason we step into the gym. Getting a pull-up or ten or a two-hundred-pound squat is not the motivation. We start because we want to look better. We want to be firmer and tighter and be able to put on that bikini and be proud and confident wearing it. Yet most women steer clear of the weight room and beeline straight to step class, because they fear that by lifting heavy things they will start to look like Ms. Olympia.

Nothing could be farther from the truth.

This is such a common fear among many women who are just stepping into fitness–that lifting heavy will produce big, bulky, and masculine muscles.

If you lift heavy weight, your body will respond and you will build muscle in line with your genetics and body structure. Your body will develop only as it can.

The number one reason you won't get big is because of testosterone.

Both men and women produce testosterone naturally; however, women produce about 1/15th the amount men do. We simply don't have the level of testosterone necessary to support a big and bulky phsyique. There is no amount of heavy lifting you can do that will get you to look "that way" without focused and consistent training, eating, and supplementing with hormones. The female bodybuilders you're thinking of right now have specifically trained to look like that for years and years; it didn't happen overnight. Gaining muscle isn't easy!

2.5 BUILDING ENERGY SYSTEMS

METABOLIC CONDITIONING

Any time you run, ride a bike, swim, jog, or even walk, you are doing some type of "cardio." You are using energy produced by the body with the foods you eat to fuel your activity. Metabolic conditioning, or metcons for short, is simply another form of cardio. The difference is how it is applied.

Cardio is synonymous with long hours on a treadmill, stair climber, or stationary bike. It's aerobic training, and it allows you to engage in low-power, extended efforts, all while decreasing body fat. The only problem with this is that it's been shown to decrease muscle mass, strength, speed, and power. **Aerobic activity burns muscle. Not what we want!**

Metabolic conditioning, on the other hand, involves short and intense bursts of exercise that can be far superior for fat loss and at the same time improve strength, muscle mass, power, speed, and endurance.

It builds both aerobic and anaerobic capacity. Anaerobic activity builds muscle. Just think—physique of marathon runner or sprinter? A-ha...hello, sprinter! Plus, it's more enjoyable and easier to stick with. Short and fast instead of thirty-minute treadmill sessions, yes please!

How does it work? How does the body get energy during exercise?

Metabolic conditioning increases your body's ability to transport oxygen from the lungs to the cells, and generates energy so you can move more efficiently. It also causes a larger metabolic response in the body, which burns more calories and raises the metabolic rate.

A really quick but important science lesson: There are three primary energy systems that the body uses for different activities.

- **The ATP-PC (phosphagen) system.**
  This is an anaerobic (without oxygen) system that produces energy very quickly but for a very short time, less than ten seconds. It would be used, for example, during a twenty-metre sprint, a near maximal lift at the gym, or a single jump. It first uses any ATP stored in the muscles, and then uses creatine phosphate (CP). Because it's so quick and powerful, it takes around two to five minutes to fully recover.

- **The Anaerobic Glycolitic, or lactic acid, system.**
  As soon as you start any high-intensity activity, you're using the anaerobic (without oxygen) glycolitic system. It creates energy exclusively from carbohydrates, with lactic acid being a by-product. It dominates in events lasting up to ninety seconds, including a weight-training set at the gym or a

400-800-metre run before muscle pain, burning, and fatigue set in, and it's difficult to keep the same intensity. Picture running really fast and then your energy dropping about 50%. That's the anaerobic glycolitic system at work. Recovery is between one and four minutes.

- **The aerobic system.**
The aerobic system (with oxygen) generates energy from the breakdown of carbohydrates and fat in the presence of oxygen so it can be kept up for longer. This energy system can go on for hours and hours of easy to moderate intensity work and it can recover in a matter of seconds. Think marathon runner.

Your body is always using all three systems. When you train, each system is contributing to some degree. The key difference between the three pathways is that the aerobic system is the only one that needs oxygen from the lungs to generate more energy. The other two are not sustainable over a long period of time, but essential for movement. For example, sprinters and powerlifters rely on anaerobic energy. Their muscles explode into activity very quickly, but the stored energy is used up pretty quick.

Metabolic conditioning is training to prompt your body to become more efficient at all forms of metabolism.

Long hours on a treadmill, stair master, or elliptical will do wonders for improving your aerobic system and cardiovascular fitness, but it won't do much to improve your phosphagen and glycolitic pathways.

The best way to train this is to use compound anaeorbic exercises combined with short, intense bursts of aerobic exercises with rest times in between.

FOCUS ON LARGE MUSCLE GROUPS

Compound movements require a maximum amount of energy, because multiple joints are involved. Squats, presses, bench presses, and pull-ups are examples of exercises that can be metabolically taxing. Runs of varying distances, sprinting, and basic gymnastics exercises such as pull-ups, pushups, and air squats, rows, dips, and high-rep Olympic lifting movements should all be included in the workouts. The Airdyne and rowing machines are great as well.

TRAIN AT HIGH INTENSITY

Metabolic training is anaerobic exercise done at high intensity. It should make you breathless.

If you're not breathing hard, you're not doing it right.

Now, this doesn't mean you have to be reaching for the puke bucket every workout. It's not about pushing your body to its limits, it's about pushing past your comfort zone. Visualize going to 80% of your intensity during your workout, whatever that may be for you. On some workouts, picture 90%, and then on occasion go all out at 100%. **Vary the intensity, but it make so that you want to come back for more.** If all you do is crazy, 100%-intense metabolic workouts all the time, your body will not be able to recover properly.

FEEL THE BURN

Don't be afraid of it! You should be feeling your muscles while you are working out. When you feel your muscles burn during a workout, you know you're creating a favourable hormonal response in your body.

DO INTERVAL TRAINING

Training intervals means exercising at different levels of intensity with rest periods in between. Intervals train both the anaerobic and aerobic system, and can include many exercises. This can include sprinting, running, jogging, walking, biking, rowing. Here's an example.

30 On/30 Off: 30 seconds of hard work, followed by 30 seconds of rest, for 10 rounds

DO TABATA TRAINING

20 seconds of hard work 10 seconds off repeated 8 times.

This may not seem like a lot work, but imagine doing this at the same intensity as Usain Bolt doing 100m sprints, and repeat. Again, the best exercises are those that involve compound movements. Squats, lunges, deadlifts, running, rowing, pull-ups, sit-ups and pushups are all great exercises. If you want to add weight, include kettlebells. All you need is a timer. Your score is your lowest number of reps performed in any of the eight sets, and your goal is to improve that next time.

DO CIRCUIT TRAINING

The great thing about circuit training is that is can be done anywhere. **Circuit training involves moving from exercise to exercise with little or not rest in between.** There are usually around ten to twelve exercises that are each done for a set time (usually about one to two minutes) or a set number of reps, before moving on

> The great thing about circuit training is that is can be done anywhere.

to the next exercise.

The great thing about circuit training is that is can be done any-where. It doesn't require expensive equipment, it can be added into a beginner's weight-training routine, it can be an amazing full-body workout, and it's an excellent way to lose inches.

CROSSFIT FILTHY 50

Do 50 repetitions of everything for time.

BOX JUMP
JUMPING PULL-UPS
KETTLE BELL SWINGS
WALKING LUNGES
KNEES TO ELBOWS
PUCH PRESS
BACK EXTENSIONS
WALL BALL SHOTS
BURPEES
DOUBLE UNDERS

The key to getting fitter is to always push yourself to work harder—to do more, to lift more. As soon as one meta-bolic pathway fails, your body slows down. By improving these ear-ly, you may speed up your fitness progress, lose weight faster, and perform better at your sport.

RECOVERY

Rest and recovery are essential to building a strong and healthy body. Before any progress is made, you have to give yourself a break. When you stress your body, it needs proper time to heal. Rest is so important for staying injury free and for setting yourself up for success. You want to be training for the long haul.

- **Get some sleep!**
  Your sleep is just as important to your health as nutrition and fitness. It gives your body time to repair muscles, build protein, create new tissue and replenish. My sleep is vital to me. If I don't get enough of it, everything suffers. Create a dark, quiet space at night. Total darkness. Cover the windows and put something over your alarm clock. Routine is everything–pick a time to go to bed and stick with it. Learn to relax and unwind.

> Before any progress is made, you have to give yourself a break.

I make sure to get at least eight hours of uninterrupted sleep every night. When I get enough sleep, my memory is sharper, I have more energy, and my body is more capable to do everyday things.

- **Play and have fun!**
  I remember playing outside as a kid until the streetlights came on. Running around all day, playing at the park with my friends, throwing the ball around the court we lived in, riding my bike, or skipping endless hours. Being active was effortless, it was fun!

As we get older, though, playtime seems to disappear. Life gets in the way, right? We forget how to play!

If you want to be a healthy person, you have to make movement a part of life every single day. Exercise doesn't always have to be regimented and organized, it can come in many forms.

The next time you groan about hitting the gym, remember what you did as a kid, how you moved your body in a way that you loved. Find other activities that you enjoy and that make you want to move, whether it's dancing, riding your bike, or going for a walk by the river. Think back to that time in your life when playing was instinctively the best use of your energy, and get out there and move!

2.6 FINDING YOUR INNER ATHLETE

You are an athlete! This is one I struggled with for quite some time. My visions of an athlete were connected to the greats like Michael Jordan or Nadia Comenici and the Olympic games. If I wasn't a pro or wasn't competing, how could I possibly be an athlete? Me?

Even after years of consistently training, saying I am an athlete seemed so foreign at times. It took me a while to accept this new identity and to be able to confidently say this and not feel like a fraud. It took a while to understand that I didn't have to win any medals or even step on a podium to be an athlete.

I just had to make a choice, and that choice was to consistently work towards health and wellness. That includes strength, fitness, nutrition, rest, recovery, and a balanced lifestyle.

Whether or not you've competed in sports, there is an athlete inside of you.

> Whether or not you've competed in sports, there is an athlete inside of you.

Even if you've never stepped foot in a gym, done a pull-up or a pushup, run a marathon or picked up a tennis racket, you have that drive within you to reach your full potential. It means you have it within you to be your best. You deserve it!

The thing is, the more I started to move, the more athletic I started to feel. I became more committed to going to the gym and eating well. **My lifestyle choices became more focused, and I started to organize my life around fitness, because it just felt so effing good!**

Finding my inner athlete has made it possible to make this a lifestyle change and not a summer season or News Year's resolution. The funny thing is, somehow in the mix I noticed I was doing all the things that "athletes" do—and I was home.

Aristotle once said, "We are what we repeatedly do. Excellence, then, is not an act, but a habit."

Make a choice. While you may never compete at a pro level, mirroring the habits of amazing athletes will help you get in better shape, improve your performance, and help you create a body and a life that you love. **You've got it inside you already!**

HERE ARE SOME TIPS FOR ACCESSING YOUR INNER ATHLETE:

- **Train for performance, not just aesthetics.**
  This was a big one for me. Most of us initially hit the gym in hopes of getting a leaner, sexier physique, and not to rip out twenty pull-ups or get a 250-pound deadlift. Those are all

very valid goals; however, it wasn't until I focused on my performance that I started to build a body that I really loved. It also helped to get rid of the psychological issues I had with body image. Instead on focusing on what I physically didn't like about my body...ugh, um, my thighs...I began to pay more attention to how my body moved and what it was capable of. Not only did I get stronger and healthier, I increased muscle mass and decreased body fat. **When you train like an athlete, performance increases and aesthetics somehow take care of themselves.**

- **Train for Strength.**
There are over 600 muscles in your body that help you to move. The stronger the muscles, the faster you run, the higher you jump, the harder you hit and further you throw. The stronger you are the more powerful you are. And an added bonus, athletes who strength train have fewer injuries. It strengthens muscle attachments and increases bone density.

- **Fuel your body the right way.**
Eating the right foods will not only give you more energy during your workouts and improve your performance, it will make you feel better and be healthier all day, every day. Make sure you are getting enough protein to help your muscles grow and the right carbohydrates and fats to give you the energy you need. And don't forget to hydrate—drink your water!

- **Rest and recover.**
Your body needs time to repair itself. Athletes take their recovery just as seriously as their training. They understand the importance of sleep, post workout nutrition, mobility, stretching and mental recovery. Muscles are built while at rest when the

body is allowed to heal itself.

- **Set goals.**
To get success, you need to set some short-term and long-term goals. Set yourself up for success. Keep track of progress and celebrate your wins. Your goals can be performance or habit based. A performance-based goal may be achieving a certain amount of reps on a workout, or a certain weight on a bar, or it may be getting your first pull-up! A habit-based goal may be as simple as committing to getting to the gym three times a week. Athletes do this on a regular basis—it ensures continual progress.

GOAL SETTING

S	SPECIFIC
M	MEASURABLE
A	ATTAINABLE
R	RELEVANT
T	TIME-BOUND

- **Envision success.**
I remember reading an interview with a famous Olympic athlete who was asked how it felt to win the gold medal. She said it felt exactly as she had felt and seen in her mind a million times. Athletes often visualize success before it even happens. They

play it over and over in their minds. Visualize what you want to achieve, be clear, and believe that it is possible!

- **Work with coaches.**
Athletes often have many coaches. Coaches help you stay focused and to keep you progressing. A strength coach can help you design programs specifically tailored to you, or a nutrition coach can help to make sure you're on track with your goals. They take away the planning so that you don't have to think about the workout, you just do it. They are also great at helping to keep you accountable.

When I first started building my body into a strong one, it started with working my muscles. I could feel the strength growing every time I left the gym. It very quickly turned to an emotional and mental strength, and as I got stronger, I began to feel more powerful, even when I was supposed to be at my weakest. Seeing what my body was truly capable of gave me the confidence to make changes in every area of my life. The same power can be yours, if you want it to be.

PART 3 :: MIND - YOUR THOUGHTS CREATE YOUR REALITY

3.1 YOU ARE AMAZING!

Admit it. If you really sat down and thought about what your body does on a regular basis every day, you would be in awe. It's constantly changing and growing. From the minute you were born up until this point, your body has replaced millions of cells. Every second of the day, your body is working through circulation, respiration, digestion, and repair without even a single conscious intention from your brain. It just happens. How incredible is that?

Unfortunately, oftentimes—as in my case—it takes some type of catastrophe like a disease or a brush with death for some of us to realize that our bodies weren't so bad to begin with. We spend so much time worrying about the size of our legs and butts that we forget how wonderful, beautiful, strong, and capable our bodies really are. We often strive for perfection, looking to others and wanting what they have—thinner legs, stronger thighs, a smaller butt, bigger boobs or smaller boobs—instead of loving what we have in this moment. We don't listen, and we ignore the needs of our bodies because we're way to busy hating them instead of loving them.

It's time to become aware and conscious that the choices you make and the thoughts that you think determine your health, physically, emotionally, and mentally. You really do have the capability to create and live your life as you desire, and your potential is limitless. It's time to **start connecting to your body and making choices that will allow you to thrive and live a long and healthy life.**

You can do this! I know you can. I've seen it over and over again. Women who start at the gym and can barely lift fifty pounds or do a pull-up and months later are lifting a hundred pounds over their heads and multiple pull-ups are no longer an issue. I've seen women lose over a hundred pounds and keep the weight off. I've seen people reverse allergies and autoimmune issues by changing their diets and focusing on eating nutritious foods. I've seen women, including myself, thrive after cancer by becoming aware, learning and applying and practicing self-love and connecting their minds and bodies. I truly believe you have the power to achieve everything that you desire, that you have power over your life and your choices.

You are not only capable of becoming strong and healthy–you deserve to be. It is who you are. Believe you can and you will.

3.2 THE POWER OF AWARENESS

> "It is our choices, Harry, that show what we truly are, far more than our abilities."
>
> J.K. Rowling, *Harry Potter and the Chamber of Secrets*

If you take a good look at the world around you, you may notice that most people are running on auto pilot. People have become really good at running through daily life without an awareness of what they are doing or why; they are just *doing*.

It's almost like learning how to drive. When you first got into that car, you were aware of each movement, you were totally present for the task at hand, both hands on the wheel, checking each mirror at the appropriate time. After a few weeks, though, it became effortless. You were able to drive, change the radio station, put your lipstick on, and check your phone (don't do that!), all with very little awareness.

How often have you said you want to be healthy and live a long life, but your behavior is totally opposite. You know you want that amazing, strong body, yet you grab for that box of cookies and eat the whole bag in one sitting. (I've done it a few times myself!) You become conditioned by events, the media, and other people around you.

Start becoming aware of your choices. Self-awareness is seeing the truth about your behavior and not listening to the excuses you may tell yourself. It's understanding your own beliefs, thoughts, and motivations, and recognizing how they affect everything you do.

When you become more self-aware, you instinctively begin to see aspects of your personality and behavior that you didn't notice before. And understanding your behavior is the first step to changing it. Be mindful. Through greater self-awareness, you become empowered to choose your own way. You get rid of auto-pilot and you consciously make better choices long before an emotional reaction or any destructive behavior.

In order to become more aware, you have to start to learn to observe. Be a witness to every act that you do and every thought that you think.

SELF-REFLECTION

To develop awareness, you have to be conscious of what is going inside you and realize it. You have to put the time in. It's not something you will find the answer to in a book, it is something that is achieved with introspection. **It's the ability to look within**

yourself and think through an action. Ask yourself questions:

"What do I really want?"

"What am I trying to achieve?"

"I want a healthy and amazing body, why do I keep sabotaging myself?"

"Why do I drink so much?"

"Why don't I feel like I am capable of all that I desire?"

Really get honest with yourself. Most people don't ever ask themselves these questions, and they often don't look at themselves for the answers. They instead play the blame game, blaming others, their environment, media, the way they were raised, and so many other external circumstances so as not to feel guilty. Look for answers within to develop a more positive approach to life.

PAY ATTENTION TO YOUR EMOTIONS

Learn to watch and observe your emotions and your feelings. Analyze them. Why did they happen? How often do you feel this way, and what actions do they lead to?

For example, here's a pretty common situation: You get into an argument or are annoyed and upset with someone or even yourself. You come home and grab the tub of Ben and Jerry's, a spoon, and sit in front of the TV, ready to devour the whole delicious thing. This will make everything better—or will it? Now's the perfect time to stop and observe.

Being aware will allow you to ask questions before you dig in. **Being aware will give you the right to choose whether you**

let your emotions dictate what happens, so you either end up licking every last drop of ice cream, or you understand that it's just your feelings that are driving your actions. You can choose to not lick the spoon dry. It may be hard, I'm not denying that, but you have the choice. You have the power to decide!

Your feelings are the same things as your energy. The specific energy you put out is what you will get back. Start to choose to feel differently than you do now, and you will experience a new world.

BE AWARE OF YOUR BODY

Pay attention to how you feel physically. How do you feel after eating a huge meal of pasta and bread? What about a great steak with a plate full of veggies? How do you feel after exercising? Do you feel better when you take longer breaks? How much sleep is enough for you to feel energized? When do you feel the most energized? Learn to listen to your body and give it what it needs.

JOURNAL

Take fifteen to twenty minutes out of your day, every day, to journal and write down what you want to achieve and change in your life. Write down everything that you are grateful for and include how you feel. Becoming more aware and conscious requires that we pay more attention. Keeping a journal is an amazing way to do this.

MEDITATE

Okay, this one here is super hard for me. It's one that I'm starting to work on more and more. I really do find it very difficult to sit still and control my thoughts. My mind just races, but I am consciously working on it, even though right now I'm so not good at it. If I'm lying in a yoga class or even at home just quiet and thinking, within about two minutes I'm already thinking about jumping up and ripping out some pull-ups or some clean and jerks.

But I understand the importance of meditation. Getting quiet, even if it's only for five minutes to start, is really therapeutic, and it allows you to become consciously aware of every moment and action.

> You have the ability and the power to create a better life for yourself, and it starts with becoming aware.

MAKE IT FUN

Create a list of things that make you feel good fast. For me it's hugging or playing with my kids, going for a hike in the forest, having a great workout at the gym, or indulging in some dark chocolate.

What choices can you make right now that will help you get more aware and closer to what you really want in life? Awareness allows you to make deliberate decisions and be guided by your mind and what makes sense instead of emotions and instincts.

You have the ability and the power to create a better life for yourself, and it starts with becoming aware.

KNOWLEDGE IS POWER

Learning about yourself and your body is the only way to health. There is no magic cure, special diet, supplement, or pill that will get you there. There are no shortcuts. What there is, is knowledge and information and action. If you want to live the healthiest version of your life, you have to inform yourself and choose to take that information and apply it every day.

That's the key: **You must apply what you learn**. You can continue to read and study and take course after course, but without practicing, you will never achieve the results you want. You have to go out and get it. That means going to the farmers' market and buying the vegetables, and setting aside time to prepare healthy and nutritious meals. It means consciously deciding to eliminate foods that you know are not providing what you need to build the strongest, healthiest you. It means packing your bag and committing to going to the gym even when you don't want to.

Creating a healthy life is not about depriving yourself. It's about treating your body with kindness and respect and giving it what it needs and deserves. And it's understanding that change takes time.

You've spent a lifetime living with certain beliefs, thoughts, actions, and motivations. Be patient with yourself as you start on this new path. Know that there will be challenges and hiccups and that if you keep pushing through, keep learning, and keep applying what you learn, you will get there. **Be patient, be determined and be consistent!**

I want you to live in the strongest, and healthiest body that you can, and I know that it is possible for you!

BEING CONSISTENT

We all know that being consistent is essential to making a change in your life. **To create a healthy life, longevity, and a strong body, a consistent routine is necessary.** Going to the gym and having a long, amazing workout once a month is very different and not as effective as doing smaller or shorter workouts three to four times a week.

Similarly, making small changes in what you eat over a longer period of time will ensure success. If you can consistently strive to make healthy choices even 50% of the time, you're on your way to positive change. Once you get to 80% or 90%, you're laughing, it becomes second nature.

The most difficult part of any accomplishment, though, is getting started. And continually trying to start something over and over again takes a lot energy. If you take time off from pursuing your goal, you will have to use all that energy to start again. If, though, you do a little bit everyday, you will carry over that energy. Have you ever gotten a gym membership, only to use it once a week or less? Doesn't it feel like you're starting over each time? Staying consistent requires less effort mentally and physically in the long run.

It also builds momentum. A body in motion tends to stay in motion!

As you consistently work toward your goals you will create a momentum that will make things happen quicker and with less effort.

You can start simple by making a choice to be consistent. Slowly improve where you are right now, and keep at it. It could be as easy as committing to get to the gym one extra day a week and doing it.

Or it could be deciding not to eat sugar for a period of ten days. So instead of eating sugar, drink water in its place, or instead of the processed sugar, eat an apple.

After the ten days, re-evaluate. See how you feel—do you have more energy? Are you enjoying the positive changes you've made? If it's a yes, add another healthy choice. Instead of burger, have some grilled fish, or go for a walk after dinner. Keep moving towards your focus, keep your mind engaged, and be consistent with your choices.

If you get off track, get right back on and start moving forward again. We are all human, and from time to time we need to refocus. Don't beat yourself up over it; just start again.

Creating a healthy, happy, loving, and amazing body and life is a journey. It's a learning process, and it doesn't happen overnight. It takes time to evolve and build a strong and healthy body. If you've committed to consistent progress toward your goal, you will start to see results and you will eventually get there. Consistency will help you succeed!

3.3 CULTIVATING LOVE

LEARNING TO LOVE YOURSELF

In my teens and twenties, I had little self-esteem. I was unsure of who I was, I didn't understand my value, and my self-worth was really non-existent. I was always trying to impress everyone around me, plagued with self-doubt and major feelings of not being good enough. I always had something to prove. Being just me was never enough.

I was very unhappy with who I was, and it played out in all of my relationships, including the one with myself. I would end up rebelling against everyone, drinking way too often to escape my reality—I thought I was more fun to be around when I wasn't actually myself. *Who would want to be around me? I'm not fun, I'm boring and quiet with not much to say. I'm not articulate enough, my memory's horrible, I'm not a good storyteller, and I'm definitely not interesting enough.* These are the stories I would tell myself all day long, my inner dialogue. I was always wishing to be more outgoing, fun, smarter, cooler, stronger. I was always wishing to be anyone but who I was.

Then I got cancer, and reflecting on it years later, it doesn't really surprise me. My cancer has been my wake-up call. It's been my reminder and my lesson that I needed to love and value myself wholly and completely—all of me—before I could create anything meaningful in my life. I've learned that everything and every relationship that I experience is directly connected to how much love I have for myself—all of me, head to toe, mind and body.

> Before anybody could treat me with the respect and love that I desired, I had to love and respect myself.

Before anybody could treat me with the respect and love that I desired, I had to love and respect myself.

You don't have to get sick to change your life. Loving yourself first is the core of joy, happiness, self-empowerment, well being, and your ability to create a life that you love. This all impacts how you think of yourself emotionally, physically, mentally, and spiritually. If you hate yourself, your body, or who you are, it's not easy to feel good.

If your body is healthy, you are able to listen to what it needs. You recognize your individual strengths and qualities and relish in the things that make you feel good way beyond the weight on the scale or that need for the "perfect body." Beauty, health, and strength come in many shapes and sizes!

Here are my favorite "exercises" to strengthen your love for the most important person in your life...YOU!

- **Pay attention to that inner voice.**
  I think most of us would be shocked if we heard a recording of our inner dialogue. So often, we treat ourselves far worse than we would treat anyone else in our lives. Your words are powerful! Be kind and gentle and patient with yourself. Talk to yourself as a loving mother would talk to her child. Praise, encourage, and support yourself every single day!

- **Spend some time alone.**
  That's right, spend the day by yourself! Meditate, go for a walk, a movie, the park, or lunch or dinner (pick the best table and enjoy it all on your own). This may feel totally uncomfortable at first. You might feel like everyone is staring at you, judging you, and wondering why you're by yourself, but they're most likely admiring the fact that you are okay at being with just you! Alone time is necessary to build your sense of self, and the more you do, the more you'll love it!

- **Value your own opinion.**
  Don't judge or criticize yourself. Your thoughts and opinions matter. Believe in yourself and don't apologize for your interests. Not everyone is going to like everything. It's okay if you like country music, don't want to party till four a.m., or love reading cheesy romance novels! Be genuine, be you, be quirky. What other people think does not matter!

- **Write yourself a love letter.**
  When you're in a new relationship, writing a love letter can be exciting, exhilarating, and passionate, and it's always full

  of love. Why not write yourself a letter, one that you'd want to receive? It doesn't have to be long, it could be as easy as "I love you" or "Dear (Insert Your name), you are amazing. I am so happy that you are a part of my life." Tell yourself everything you love about you. Read it to yourself every day, write in your mirror, leave it on your fridge. Begin a romance with yourself!

- **Move your body.**
  Get out for a walk, go the gym, do a yoga class, take a hike! Learn about nutrition and how different foods provide optimum energy and clarity. **Cherish your body, it's amazing!**

- **Don't play small.**
  There is only one you, and you're here to show the world your uniqueness. **Shine your light bright!** You are amazing!

LOVE YOUR BODY

This topic, I think, can be a book on its own. Every day and in so many ways, the media, society, and the beauty industry tell women and girls that in order to be admired and desired they have to have the perfect body. Thin hips, lean legs, the perfect boobs, and NO cellulite. How realistic is this? Stretch marks, cellulite, birthmarks, scars, wrinkles—these are all part of each and every one of us. They make up who we are, what we've been through...they help us tell our story.

I honestly don't know one single woman who has not struggled internally with how she looks. Not one who hasn't compared herself to society's ideal and at some point felt less than. Not one who hasn't wished to look like that fitness model on the cover of a magazine.

I believe that every woman deserves to feel beautiful,

and your body does not define that beauty.

Body image and feelings about yourself are not always easy to change, but there are things that you can do to help you SHIFT YOUR FOCUS!

- **Stop dieting!**
  Yes, you heard me right. There a millions of ads targeting diets as being the secret to weight loss; it's a billion-dollar industry. Instead, start learning about nutrition and which foods will help you create a healthy body, the foods that will make you thrive.

- **Knowledge is power!**
  When you catch yourself criticizing your body or what you've eaten, stop and remind yourself that this exact thinking is part of the problem. Stop the self-loathing and embrace your uniqueness. Look to see the good, not the "bad." Perfection is not attainable. You will mess up, and that's okay! Start again and don't feel bad about it!

- **Celebrate your body!**
  Spend time being in awe at the amazing and wonderful things your body is capable of.

- **Stop reading magazines that promote an unhealthy body image.**
  Most of these girls have been airbrushed, Photoshopped, or made up with so much makeup that is distorts the reality of what they actually look like.

- **Get rid of your scale!!!**
  You don't need it!

- **Do some mirror work.**
  Look at yourself in the mirror daily naked and tell yourself how beautiful you are. It may feel strange at first, but it will get easier and eventually even fun. Focus on the parts of you that you're most critical of and keep telling yourself how amazing you are!

- **Move. Move. Move and then move some more!**
  Start connecting with your body on a regular basis. Get off the couch or the office chair and walk. Take the stairs, not the elevator. Park your car at the opposite end of the parking lot. Lift some weight, get strong!

- **Remind yourself that you are unique.**
  There is no other person on this Earth that is like you and YOU ARE SEXY! All of you!

3.4 GETTING CONNECTED

More and more people are becoming aware of the mind-body connection these days, although it's not a new concept at all. Your connection to both mind and body is so important to your self-awareness. **Everything is connected!**

Let's just take a look at our bodies. If your mouth waters at the thought of eating something fantastic, that's mind-body connection. Have you ever felt butterflies in your stomach as you were about to speak in front of a crowd, or have you seen someone in freeze in their tracks out of fear? It's all connected.

Your body is influenced by your mind, and your mind is influenced by all the hormones in your body, and your emotions are influenced by the way you care for your body! If you take care of your physical self, your mind will benefit—and vice versa.

How you treat yourself, the choices you make about your food and drink, and how you move are all connected to how you feel throughout the day, and will ultimately effect the kind of life you have!

The great thing about this is that this connection already exists inside you–you were born with it. You may not be aware or conscious of it on a daily basis, but it's there. The more you start to listen to your body, the more you will understand how what you eat an how you move effect your life. Many people ignore the way they feel, and their bodies end up screaming at them in the form of illness, disease, depression, or weight gain. Learning to listen to your body, connecting what you think and how you feel is so important. Your body wants you to survive. Listen to your body and give it what it needs!

LEARN TO TRUST YOUR GUT

Yes, you should learn how to trust your gut. We all have that sixth sense or intuition that helps guide us to make faster and smarter choices, though we often let our rational thinking override it. It's that feeling you get in the bottom of your stomach when something pops up and you have a choice you need to make. It can either loud and clear, like it's screaming at you, or subtle–a gentle nudge. Sometimes it's a feeling of calm, a "don't worry, everything will be okay," feeling. **Whatever it is, your intuition gives you guidance, so learn to listen!**

When I found that lump in my breast, I was told on so many occasions by different doctors that it was nothing, that young women have lumpy breasts. My gut was screaming at me to have it taken out anyway. So I did despite what I was advised. That digging, that deep-down feeling, was the deciding factor.

There are a few ways that you can get clearer on what your gut is trying to tell you. The first is to get quiet and clear your mind of any chatter. **Focus on what your gut is telling you and trust that it's guiding you in the right direction.** Listen to your body. The other is to think of a positive time in your life and remember the feeling associated with that time, and then think of a negative experience and recall those feelings. Now pick a current situation and pay attention to the feelings that come up. Don't judge them. Are the feelings closer to the positive or negative experience in your life? Whatever the answer is, start paying attention to your instincts and just notice.

> Nourish your body, move on a daily basis, and take steps to consistently improve your mindset.

This might not even surprise you, as instinctually you do this all the time. You may find this amazingly helpful, though, if you spend more time in head and ignore your feelings. You can never go wrong if you listen to your gut! **It's called honouring your choices and your decisions, and it's one of the most important things you can do.**

A FINAL NOTE

Remember that what's important is not how you look, it's how you feel—and you have so much control over how you feel.

It's about how I feel when I give my body what it needs to thrive. When I'm disciplined and connected and focused on my goals. When I'm doing everything I can to make my body and mind feel it's best, feeding my body nourishing foods, moving my body and getting it strong, sleeping and connecting to my inner self.

The whole goal of this book is to inspire you to make changes in your life that stay for long run. It's not a quick fix or a short-term plan.

It's a journey into developing a healthy body that will help you take action in creating a life of your dreams. It's about creating a confidence in yourself by learning to care, love and respect yourself.

Good health and a strong body start with awareness and develop with consistent action. They're personal responsibilities in making the right choices for you and your goals. They require a discipline and desire to make changes in your life; a daily commitment. You have to want health, and you have take action to get it, and I promise you it is yours for the taking. Remember, knowledge is power. I hope what you've learned here will help you to start on your path to a strong and healthy life, one where you thrive!

Don't forget that it takes time for change—it doesn't happen overnight. It's important to start now, be kind and supportive to yourself.

Encourage yourself to keep going, even if you mess up and have to start again. Continually improve the choices that you make. Nourish your body, move on a daily basis, and take steps to consistently improve your mindset. Your body is the vehicle that takes you through this amazing life. Love yourself, be kind to yourself, respect yourself, and, most importantly, believe you can.

You are amazing!

Gordana J

xo

References:

William & Devlin, 1992; Williams, 1998; Tarnpolsky et al., 1992; Lemon et al., 1992.

The Definitive Guide to Saturated Fat (Mark's Daily Apple)

Precious Yet Perilous: Understanding the Essential Fatty Acids (Weston A. Price Foundation)

Metabolism and Ketosis (Michael Eades)

http://ajcn.nutrition.org/content/75/5/951.2.full Is dietary carbohyrdate essential for human nutrition? 2002 American Society for Clinical Nutrition

http://www.jissn.com/content/4/1/8. International Society of Sports Nutrition position stand: protein and exercise. 2007 Journal of the international society of sports nutrition.

Cordain, L. Cereal Grains: Humanity's Double-Edged Sword in Simopoulos, AP (ed): Evolutionary Aspects of Nutrition and Health. DIet, Exercise, Genetics, and Chronic Disease. World Review of Nutrition and Deitetics, vol. 84, 1999.

The Argument Against Cereal Grains (Kurt Harris, MD)

Living with Phytic Acid (Weston A. Price Foundation)

Scritinizing Soy (Marks Daily Apple)

Dairy: food of the Gods or neolithic agent of disease? (Chris Kresser)

Dairy: 6 Reasons You Should Avoid It at All Costs or WHy Following the USDA Food Pyramid Guidelines is Bad for Your Health (VIDEO) (Mark Hyman, MD)

A Comparison Between Human Milk and Cows Milk (Viva Health)

On Dairy and Insulin (Marks Daily Apple)

Erasmus, Udo. Fats that Heal Fats that Kill. Summertown, TN. Alive Books. 1993.

Donnelly, JE, et al. 2004. The role of exercise for weight loss and maintenance. Best Pract Res Clin Gastroenterol. (http://www.ncbi.nlm.nih.gov/pubmed/15561636)

Haas, Elson M. and Buck Levin. Staying Healthy with Nutrition. The Complete Guide to Diet and Nutritional Medicine. Berkely, CA. Celestial Arts. 2006. p.25.

http://www.nichd.nih.gov/health/topics/bonehealth/conditioninfo/Pages/activity.aspx

Marieb, Elaine N. Essentials of Human Anatomy & Physiology. 9th Ed. San Francisco, CA. 2009.

http://www.marksdailyapple.com/case-against-cardio/#axzz37xDptYCd A Case Against Cardio (from a former mileage king) (Marks Daily Apple)

Bean, Anita. The Complete Guide to Sports Nutrition. 7th ed. London. Bloomsbury. 2013.

www.ingramcontent.com/pod-product-compliance
Lightning Source LLC
Chambersburg PA
CBHW051027030426
42336CB00015B/2749